The Heart of the Matter

Questions to Ask Your Cardiologist

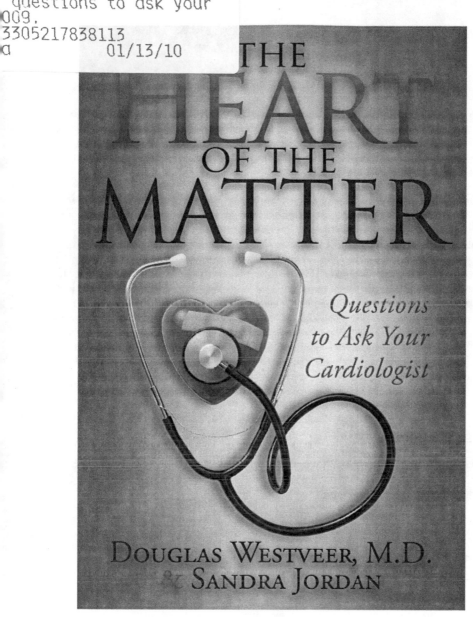

THE HEART OF THE MATTER

*Questions
to Ask Your
Cardiologist*

DOUGLAS WESTVEER, M.D.
& SANDRA JORDAN

New York

The Heart of the Matter
Questions to Ask Your Cardiologist

ISBN 978-1-60037-633-7

Library of Congress Control Number: 2009903537

Cover Design by: Rachel Lopez
　　　　　　　　rachel@r2cdesign.com

MORGAN · JAMES
THE ENTREPRENEURIAL PUBLISHER

Morgan James Publishing, LLC
1225 Franklin Ave., STE 325
Garden City, NY 11530-1693
Toll Free 800-485-4943
www.MorganJamesPublishing.com

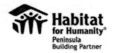

In an effort to support local communities, raise awareness and funds, Morgan James Publishing donates one percent of all book sales for the life of each book to Habitat for Humanity. Get involved today, visit **www.HelpHabitatForHumanity.org**.

Contents

Preface

Even after twenty eight years of practicing cardiology, our failure to encourage patients to advocate for their own health and safety are perplexing. As a practicing physician at Northpointe Heart Center and the cardiology division director at William Beaumont Hospital in Troy, Michigan, I've witnessed the benefits of having well informed patients. Armed with the right information, you can make a big difference in your struggle with heart disease. However, the complexity of the information available to you can be overwhelming. Therefore, every page of information entered into this book was first shared with Sandy Jordan, an educator of young children. Her insight, common sense, and continuous striving toward simplicity in the explanations and vocabulary we selected played a vital role in being sure that what we convey to you is appropriate and correct. Finally, our book is dedicated to our patients. Over the years, I have listened to your fears as you confront your disease. Ultimately, the only solution to your fear is information. We wish you the very best as you learn more about your heart.

D.C.W.

Acknowledgements

The authors are very thankful to our families who have been patient with us during the entire process of writing this book. Dr. Westveer is especially thankful to the physicians at Northpointe Heart Center who have inspired us to always provide the best possible care for our patients. We also want to thank the armies of clinical researchers in cardiology who tirelessly weave the results of clinical studies into treatment strategies that make a difference to your care. We especially acknowledge the relentless work of the American Heart Association and the American College of Cardiology and their many researchers, and highly recommend their websites to you for additional information (www.americanheart.org; www.acc.org). Dr. Westveer is also grateful to the members and leaders of the Department of Cardiology at William Beaumont Hospitals. Their passion to discover the best treatment for patients with heart disease has provided the framework to write this book. Foremost among them we acknowledge Dr. Gerald Timmis, the senior author for cardiology texts published more than two decades ago and Dr. Barry Franklin, a passionate and dedicated longtime academic leader. They have planted the seed that still drives us to educate others. We also want to thank Roberta Ancona for her invaluable assistance and never-ending support.

Introduction

Every unexpected pain in the chest is a chilling reminder of the threat posed by our nation's biggest killer: heart disease. The good news is that the incidence of cardiovascular disease is finally decreasing in our country. From 1994 to 2004, the American Heart Association reported that death rates from cardiovascular disease declined for the first time in over a century. In part, this reduction reflects better lifestyle choices as well as new treatments, medications, and interventions. Nonetheless, heart disease is still too prevalent. Nearly 2400 Americans die of cardiovascular disease each day, an average of one death every 37 seconds. Moreover, people dying of cardiovascular disease are tragically young. More than 148,000 Americans younger than 65 years of age died last year from this tragic killer. Furthermore, the four decade-long decline in heart disease may be coming to a screeching halt. Recent research found a surprisingly high incidence of serious blockages in the blood vessels of adolescents and young adults dying from accidental or homicidal death, a startling reminder that heart disease is not going away.

How can we best combat these frightening statistics? We live in an era that has seen our knowledge of medicine progress at a speed that is unprecedented in human history. Today, we can conquer illness that once seemed inevitably fatal. The progress in treating and preventing heart disease has been particularly daunting in the past 25 years, as new options to prevent and treat heart disease continue to fill our newspapers and journals on a daily basis. Understanding this progress presents serious challenges. Each month, the stack of medical journals on my desk gets closer to the ceiling. My first reaction is to blame myself for not taking enough time to work through it all. But a more thorough analysis is more alarming. The volume and complexity of investigative studies in cardiology are growing enormously. It is now estimated that the average doctor requires five years to digest all the research currently being reported every twenty-four hours. The problem is even more complex for you and your family. My patients have never been more eager to learn about their disease, but never more frustrated by the lack of meaningful and accurate resources to help them.

Inadequate access to reliable health care information is detrimental to your health! This book was written to provide insight for you and your family into this mountain of information. The book will lead you through an understanding of what you need to know about heart attacks, heart surgery, hypertension, high cholesterol, and heart failure. We'll help you understand cardiac procedures like pacemakers and defibrillators and acquaint you with the medications used to treat your heart disease. As you begin your journey, you may find your physician somewhat overwhelmed and perhaps even provoked by your informed questions. Be kind, patient, and understanding. However, if a relationship of mutual trust cannot be quickly achieved, change doctors! Effectively sharing information is time consuming and personally challenging to some physicians. Prescribing a cholesterol medication takes two minutes, but discussing the reasons to take it may consume the entire visit. Ultimately, you must wade through the data with your doctor since you will be the recipient of both the benefits and the complications of the recommendations given to you.

The recommendations in this book are derived from evidence-based scientific studies and widely adopted treatment guidelines that are complemented by years of clinical practice. We have attempted to extract from these guidelines those that are most meaningful to you, and condense them into understandable terms. At the same time, guidelines are only guidelines. For many reasons, the care of each patient must be approached individually. The book therefore also relies upon my patient interactions during 28 years of practicing clinical cardiology to help you understand what's important and what's not.

We want to remind our readers that the best medical decisions for your heart condition are complex and must be evaluated on an individual basis. We have tried hard to be complete, current, and fair in providing medical information for you. However, the best choices for your care can only be made after a thorough discussion with your doctor and a review of all of your personal information. In no way should the generalizations made in this book replace the individual decision-making necessary in your own care.

Chapter 1: The Normal Human Heart

Heart disease always relates to an abnormality in the structure or function of the normal heart. So let's begin by exploring how the normal heart works.

Q:?? How is my heart built?

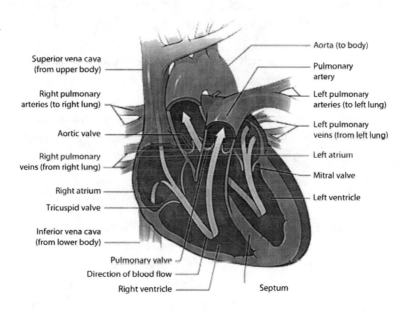

The heart is an extraordinarily dynamic organ, consisting of muscle, blood vessels, valves, and an electrical system. It is divided into four chambers. The two upper chambers are called the right and left atria. The two lower chambers are called the right and left ventricles. Figure 1 illustrates the anatomy of the normal human heart and the pattern of blood flowing through each chamber:

Q:?? How does blood flow through my heart?

Let's follow the pattern of how blood flows through our bodies by envisioning ourselves clinging to a blood cell floating through the body. The blood cells provide oxygen and other nutrients to your tissues. Once the cells have completed their task, they must return to your heart, then to the lungs to pick up more oxygen, and finally back out to your body. Figure 1 outlines for the paths that you will take as you circulate through the heart. The first leg of your trip carries you through veins, the conduits that carry all of our blood back to our heart. You enter the right atrium of the heart through either the superior vena cava from the upper part of the body or the inferior vena cava from below. From the right atrium, you flow across the tricuspid valve and into the right ventricle. The right ventricle then contracts, closing the tricuspid valve and opening the pulmonary valve. The right ventricle gives you the boost you need to cross the pulmonary valve into the pulmonary arteries on your way to the lungs. The lungs give you oxygen from the air we breathe. You then return to the heart through the pulmonary veins. Two pulmonary veins drain blood from the right lung and two from the left lung back to the left atrium. You will then cross the mitral valve and enter into the left ventricle. The left ventricle is the major pumping chamber of the heart, and pumps you across the aortic valve, out of the heart, and into the aorta. You are now traveling through conduits away from the heart called arteries. The oxygen you carry is then delivered to the tissues of the body, and the circuit of blood flow is finally completed.

Q:?? How do the heart valves work?

The heart has four valves. The purpose of each valve is to be sure that blood flows in the right direction. The right side of the heart contains the tricuspid and pulmonary valves; the left side contains the mitral and aortic valves. On the right side, the tricuspid valve needs to open to allow blood to enter into the right ventricle. Once the right ventricle has filled, it begins to contract, pumping blood towards the lungs. At this point, the tricuspid valve closes, so that blood does not leak backwards. In the same fashion, as the right ventricle contracts, the pulmonary valve must open, allowing blood to exit the right ventricle into the pulmonary artery. When the right ventricle is done pumping, the pulmonary valve closes so that blood pumped into the lungs does not leak back into the right ventricle. The same process repeats itself on the left side of the heart. The blood passes from the left atrium across the open mitral valve, which must close as the left ventricle contracts. The aortic valve then opens to allow blood to exit the heart to the body.

Q:?? How do heart valves become defective?

The heart's valves can become too stiff or too leaky. A valve that is too stiff and can't open is called a stenotic valve. One that is leaky and can't close completely is called an insufficient valve. For example, aortic stenosis is a disease that stiffens the aortic valve and prevents it from fully opening. In contrast, mitral insufficiency is a leaky mitral valve that allows blood pumped from the left ventricle to be pumped backwards into the lungs.

Coronary Arteries of the Heart

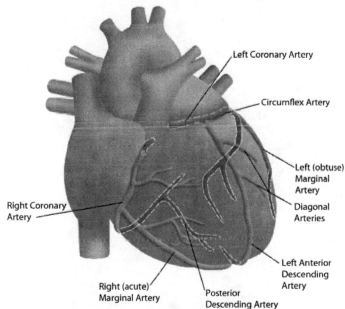

Q:?? How is my heart supplied with blood?

The blood vessels that supply the heart with its blood are called coronary arteries. Most of us have three main arteries that arise from the aorta just beyond the aortic valve.   The anatomy of the three coronary arteries is shown in Figure 2.

The coronary arteries are the first branches of the aorta.   On the right side of the aorta, the right coronary artery, or RCA, arises and travels down the right side of the heart to supply both the right and bottom surfaces.   On the left side, a short left main coronary artery (LMCA) arises that quickly divides into two branches. The front branch is called the left anterior descending artery, or LAD. The LAD supplies both the front wall of the heart and the septum, or the wall that divides the two ventricles in half. The back branch is the left circumflex artery, which travels down the back and left side of the heart. Once the blood has nourished the heart muscle, it returns to the heart through the veins, converging on a large vein call the coronary sinus. The coronary sinus dumps its blood into the right atrium. It joins the remainder of the blood returning to the heart from the rest of the body and heads out to the lungs to be replenished with oxygen.

Electrical System of the Heart

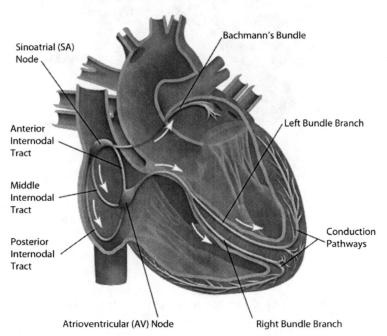

4

Q:?? What about the electrical system of the heart?

Every good pump requires an electrical system to organize all of its mechanical events. The heart consists of millions of individual heart cells, each too small to be seen by the human eye. In order for the heart to contract in a coordinated fashion and actually pump blood, each of these cells must contract at exactly the same time. It is the responsibility of the electrical system of the heart to be sure that each cell contributes to a synchronized contraction.

The heart's electrical system is illustrated in Figure 3. The electrical signals begin in the upper portion of the right atrium, in a small structure called the sinus node. The sinus node is a specialized collection of electrical cells that function like a spark plug. If you have ever gotten your finger caught in a wall plug, you know that electricity causes muscle to jump. In the heart, the spark from the sinus node is first delivered to the upper chambers causing them to contract. The impulses then converge on another specialized collection of cells halfway between the upper and lower chambers called the atrioventricular node, or AV node. Conduction of electricity is slowed somewhat through the AV node resulting in a brief pause after which electricity travels out of the AV node, again down specialized wires to the right and the left ventricles. Once again, the stimulation of electricity hitting the heart muscle in the lower chambers causes the lower chambers to contract. In this way, the heart has a coordinated contraction, beginning with the atrial contraction and followed by the ventricular contraction. This sequence is repeated every time the heart beats. As we exercise, the sinus node picks up its rate of stimulation and the heart rate increases. As we sleep, the sinus node causes the heart rate to decrease.

Problems may arise with the electrical system of the heart. In some of us, the sinus node malfunctions, fashionably called sick sinus syndrome. In another example, the wires of the heart stop conducting electricity down to the heart muscle. This condition is called heart block. Typically, the heartbeat slows down considerably when the electrical system fails, and fatigue, shortness of breath or loss of consciousness may occur.

Chapter 2: The Diseases of the Heart

I've had a heart attack

You are not alone in your fight against heart disease. In 2007, an estimated 770,000 Americans had a new heart attack, and 430,000 additional people had a recurrent one. This amounts to a new coronary event about every 37 seconds and nearly two deaths every minute. However, good news is on the horizon. Improved treatment and better prevention are finally eating away at our risks of a heart attack. National programs to bring about these improvements are actually ahead of schedule. You need to be aware of all of the possible options available to you to treat your heart disease because your fight will make a difference!

Q:?? What is a myocardial infarction?

In medical terms, you've had a "myocardial infarction." The term "myocardial" means heart muscle, and "infarction" means death of tissue. Your myocardial infarction, or MI, occurred because a blood vessel going to your heart became obstructed with hardening of the arteries and clot. The process of how this happens is a long story with a fast final chapter. Over many years, a process that still remains incompletely understood inflamed the inner lining of your blood vessels. Inflammation causes microscopic cracks inside the blood vessel's wall. Our bodies constantly attempt to heal internal injuries, and numerous repair cells circulating through the blood stream perform much of this job. Repair cells are constantly searching out injured blood vessels, and sacrifice themselves as they patch them up. The cells accomplish their mission successfully but tragically leave behind LDL cholesterol, the major building block for these repair cells. The remnants of the repair process then form an area of hardening of the arteries called plaque. Gradually, more cholesterol, scar tissue, blood clot and other debris build up to increase the size of the plaque and narrow the vessel. Years later, the final chapter suddenly begins. In some cases, blood flow through the badly narrowed plaque becomes so severely restricted that the blood flow trickles to a halt, allowing a blood clot to form that totally obstructs the artery bringing about a heart attack. In other cases, a more recently described catastrophic event evolves called plaque rupture. In this process, the plaque buildup may not be that severe, but suddenly the tissue under the plaque bleeds and becomes acutely inflamed. Within hours, the eruption may push the plaque outward into the channel of the artery, causing sudden, severe and often complete obstruction. Plaque rupture can change an artery that is only mildly blocked to one that is totally occluded in hours or a few days. This sudden process may explain why some patients have no symptoms before a heart attack strikes.

Heart cells can only live a few hours without an adequate blood supply before heart muscle damage begins. When a severely blocked blood vessel totally obstructs, the heart muscle supplied by the blood vessel begins to rapidly die. Once the muscle dies, it is gradually replaced by scar tissue and the vitality of the heart's contraction is lost. At that point, the evolution of your heart attack is complete.

Q:?? Is my chest pain caused by a heart attack?

Symptoms of a heart attack vary substantially. Most patients describe some form of centrally located chest discomfort. Words such as pressure, tightness, heaviness, and squeezing are often used. The discomfort may be perceived in either arm, the back, or up into the throat or jaws. Although cardiac pain is more commonly felt in the left arm, it may radiate into either or both arms, or remain only in the chest. The pain may vary a lot in intensity, with some patients experiencing excruciating discomfort while others feel only mild pressure. Additional symptoms may also occur, including shortness of breath, severe fatigue, unusual sweating, or nausea.

Some patients may present with unusual symptoms restricted to vague discomfort or fatigue. Unusual symptoms from a heart attack experienced by a minority of people are called atypical symptoms.

Women and diabetics in particular often present with atypical symptoms. For this reason, we have an old saying that every pain between the nose and the navel should be considered heart pain until proven otherwise. It is far wiser to assume that your pain is coming from your heart and act accordingly than die at home with an antacid in your hand!

Q:?? Should I call 911 or drive to the hospital?

If you suspect you are having a heart attack, call 911 and be transported to your hospital as quickly as possible. Obstructed blood flow to your heart begins to damage your heart muscle within minutes, and virtually all of the damage is complete within twelve hours. If your heart damage is to be reversed, the blood flow to your heart must be re-established quickly. One of the common delays in treating heart attack victims occurs before patients ever seek medical care. Some patients refuse to acknowledge their symptoms and delay calling for help. Others lose vital minutes trying to contact their doctor. Don't delay; call EMS (emergency medical services) immediately if you are at all suspicious you are having a heart attack. Many EMS providers are now able to perform electrocardiograms in your home, drastically reducing the time necessary to diagnose a heart attack. Nitroglycerin, aspirin, and other important medications that we will review shortly can be given to you earlier by an EMS provider if you call 911. In addition, the early minutes of a heart attack have the highest incidence of lethal rhythm disturbances. No treatment for you is available if you collapse in your automobile. Only an EMS provider can deliver successful resuscitation for these threatening complications. Finally, you will more likely survive your heart attack with less heart damage if emergency, expert angioplasty is available at the hospital to which you are transported. We will discuss shortly the importance of opening an obstructed artery to save your heart by angioplasty, but first you need to get to the right hospital. Your EMS service will likely be informed about the nearest hospital capable of providing this up to date technology. It is clearly in your best interest to request that your EMS provider bypass a nearer hospital incapable of angioplasty, and transport you quickly to an angioplasty-capable facility.

Q:?? Can I survive this heart attack?

Being hospitalized with a heart attack is very serious. Nearly half of patients die suddenly or within minutes of the onset of symptoms, before access to medical care. Even with the most advanced treatment available, an additional 10 to 15% of patients die in the hospital. Two complications most commonly occur. Nearly half of patients who have a heart attack die from an abnormal rhythm disturbance arising from injury to the heart muscle. These arrhythmias usually occur before hospitalization, are immediately lethal, and result in sudden collapse and death. Even small heart attacks can be complicated by this sudden rhythm disturbance, called ventricular fibrillation. The second complication from a heart attack is heart failure resulting from excessive damage to the heart muscle. Heart failure develops more gradually, perhaps over hours following a heart attack, and is associated with significant shortness of breath, a drop in blood pressure, and insufficient blood flow to critical organs of the body such as the kidneys.

Although heart attacks are very serious, the outlook for most patients is improving rapidly. New technologies and medications have improved survival and decrease the tragic complications of heart failure, stroke, and serious abnormal rhythm disturbances. Take your disease seriously and follow your treatment plan flawlessly.

Q:?? Why is an EKG so important?

The key test to diagnose a heart attack is the electrocardiogram (EKG). One of the oldest tests in cardiology, the EKG is commonly diagnostic of a heart attack, particularly when a major blood vessel to the heart is obstructed. It is extremely important to obtain an EKG as quickly as possible after the onset of chest pain. As we will discuss momentarily, quickly opening a completely obstructed artery to the heart is crucial to minimize heart damage. The electrocardiogram is such an important tool in evaluating heart attacks that many emergency medical service personnel are now capable of performing electrocardiograms at the site where your heart attack occurs. The EKG is then transmitted by cell phone to a hospital where a team can begin preparation for your arrival. This is one of the most important reasons why calling 911 if you suspect a heart attack is a better choice than coming to the hospital by car. In any busy emergency room, delays may occur in caring for patients who appear somewhat less sick than others. However, as an advocate for your own health, insist on an EKG as quickly as possible after your arrival to the ER. Do not allow yourself to be relegated to a triage area for longer than a few moments. Be sure that a competent emergency physician quickly reviews your EKG, and ask whether your EKG is abnormal. Early diagnosis is essential to your survival.

Q:?? What are cardiac enzymes?

Particularly with a small heart attack, the EKG may only show minor changes or in fact may be entirely normal. In these circumstances, blood work to analyze for enzyme elevations may confirm that you've had a heart attack. The heart muscle cells are constantly contracting because of chemical reactions brought about by enzymes normally located inside the cells. When the heart is damaged, the enzymes spill out of the damaged cells and flood the bloodstream. Thus, a blood test showing elevation in the cardiac enzymes may be diagnostic of a heart attack. However, since enzymes may not elevate for the first 12 hours after the heart attack has started, initial treatment is often begun even when enzymes are normal. You should also be aware that other causes besides a heart attack may be responsible for elevation in the enzymes; they are not always specifically diagnostic of a heart problem.

Q:?? What testing should be done later in my hospitalization?

Following the diagnosis of a heart attack, additional testing may be necessary during your convalescent phase. Two goals are important. The amount of damage to your heart muscle must be measured. Secondly, problems with your health that may increase your risk of a future heart attack need to be identified and managed. First, what about the size of your heart attack, or the amount of muscle damage that has occurred?

Q:?? How do I find out the size of my heart attack?

The amount of heart muscle damage is often estimated by measuring the ejection fraction from the echocardiogram. In essence, the heart muscle receives incoming blood with each heartbeat, and then pumps a certain percentage of that blood out to the body. The normal heart never empties itself after beating. Rather, it normally ejects about 60% of the blood that it holds. This is your ejection fraction, or the fraction of blood ejected with each heartbeat. Heart attacks typically lower the ejection fraction due to heart muscle damage. A major heart attack may result in an ejection fraction of 30% to 40%, although ejection fractions may occasionally decrease to less than 20%. Before you go home from the hospital you should know what your ejection fraction is, since your outlook and treatment critically depend on how much damage occurred.

Following your heart attack, it is important to search for risk factors that might increase your chances of a second one in the future. For example, having blockages in coronary arteries unrelated to the one causing your heart attack significantly increases your chances of another heart attack down the road. Searching for more blockages is therefore an important plan to avoid another attack. Before you are discharged, discuss with your doctor the results of your tests that identify the condition of the blood vessel that caused your heart attack, as well as the other blood vessels supplying your heart with blood. You should also be familiar with your blood cholesterol levels and the results of any other blood or heart tests done during your hospitalization.

Q:?? Should I have a heart catheterization after my heart attack?

In some patients who have suffered a heart attack, a decision is made at the onset not to perform a cardiac catheterization to open the blocked blood vessel. Nevertheless, it is important to know whether more blockages may be present. Two strategies are often used to search for additional blockages. A "noninvasive" strategy usually involves exercise treadmill testing. A markedly abnormal exercise test suggests a higher chance for more blockages, whereas a normal response to exercise would indicate a lower chance. This approach is not perfect, but is accurate in 70% to 80% of patients capable of generating a good exercise effort. An "invasive" strategy employs cardiac catheterization to advance a small tube through an artery in the groin and into the heart. X-ray pictures are then taken of the arteries that supply the heart muscle with blood. This may have already been performed if an angiogram of the heart muscle was obtained at the time of your admission to the hospital. A heart catheterization gives more accurate information about the condition of your blood vessels, but the risk of the procedure is also slightly higher than exercise testing. The decision as to whether an invasive or noninvasive strategy is in your best interest is a very complex decision, based on your age, general health, the amount of heart muscle damage done by the heart attack, and whether additional diseases such as diabetes or hypertension are present. In most circumstances, an invasive strategy is preferred if you have recurrent chest pain following your heart attack, or if you have new EKG changes, heart failure, cardiac arrhythmias, a significantly reduced ejection fraction, or recent angioplasty in the last few months. Also, younger patients and those with risk factors that increase their chances of another heart attack are more likely to be offered an invasive approach. A noninvasive strategy may be more appropriate for older individuals with smaller, uncomplicated heart attacks, and those who have minimal or no additional risk factors for more heart attacks in the future.

If an invasive strategy is selected for you, ask about the timing of angioplasty or surgery to fix any additional blockages. Although it may seem wise to fix additional blockages quickly before they cause trouble, evidence confirms that the timing of these procedures is important to your outcome. Clearly, additional blockages should not be repaired when the blood vessel causing your heart attack is opened. Complications during such combined procedures are prohibitively high, and the time delay required to fix them in the future carries a surprisingly small risk. Whether additional blockages should be repaired towards the end of your hospitalization or after a two to four week healing period is controversial, and the timing should be approached on an individual basis after careful discussion with your doctor. In general, don't be overly concerned if a healing period of several weeks is recommended before the additional blockages are fixed.

Q:?? What about calcium scans and CT angiography?

Calcium is commonly found in the plaque that narrows our coronary arteries. It is a hard mineral that often shows up well on x-rays. A CT scan is a special x-ray that detects and quantifies the amount of calcium in our blood vessels. The results, reported as a "calcium score," range from zero in healthy arteries to over 1500 in patients with advanced blockages. The calcium score is a well-researched marker of disease and correlates with the risk of having another heart attack. The risk of a heart attack rises seven times in patients with a score between 100 and 300. Scores above 300 raise the risk of heart attack nearly ten fold. Nonetheless, if you have already had a heart attack, the added benefit of obtaining a calcium score may be limited, unless you feel that the results may make you more aggressive in reversing your risk factors.

Imaging techniques and computer speeds have improved CT scanning to the extent that blockages within some coronary arteries can now be visualized without catheterization. These scans are obtained quickly and with minimal risk. The test can predict normal coronary arteries with a high degree of accuracy, and is also fairly accurate in arteries with mild to moderate blockage and little calcium. However, predicting significant narrowing becomes less accurate as the degree of narrowing increases and particularly as more calcium begins to harden the plaque. For these reasons, catheterization may not be avoidable in some circumstances. In addition, CT scans require the injection of the same dye used in catheterization and may result in allergic reactions or kidney problems. Some researchers are also concerned about the incidence of radiation-induced cancer many years after the use of frequent CT scans, although newer technologies reduce the overall radiation exposure. The risks and benefits of CT scanning in regard to all of these issues should be discussed carefully with your doctor before choosing the best test to look at your coronary arteries.

Q:?? What test results are important to know?

As you prepare to go home from the hospital, have your doctor summarize for you the results of the following tests:
- Know your ejection fraction.
- Know your total cholesterol, HDL, LDL, and triglyceride levels.
- Know which of your three coronary arteries have blockages.
- If a stent was placed in your heart, know the kind of stent and be sure to keep the card from the manufacturer summarizing the stent information.

Treating your heart attack

Q:?? How can my obstructed blood vessel be opened?

The electrocardiogram obtained upon admission to the hospital will usually indicate whether a major blood vessel to your heart has closed. A major obstruction results in an EKG pattern called "ST elevation myocardial infarction", or STEMI, as we call it. An obstruction in a smaller artery, or an incomplete obstruction in a bigger artery results in a so called "non-ST elevation myocardial infarction", or NSTEMI. Why the difference? In most cases, a major heart attack, or STEMI, requires that the blood vessel to the heart be opened as quickly as possible. In smaller heart attacks, or NSTEMIs, a more conservative approach with medication will usually suffice.

In a STEMI heart attack, opening the obstructed coronary artery is the earliest and most important treatment strategy to save your life and preserve your heart muscle. Opening the artery allows blood flow to again nourish the area of damage. The goal of therapy is to achieve early, full, and sustained blood flow in the blocked blood vessel. Heart cells cannot live long without blood supply. Damage begins within minutes, and by 12 hours virtually all of the damage is complete and irreversible. In the management of heart attacks, minutes may determine your survival and the extent of damage to your heart. The national goal for the management of heart attacks is to reestablish blood flow through an obstructed artery within 90 minutes of your arrival to the hospital. This goal is highly aggressive, and cannot be accomplished in every patient. If available in your hospital, a balloon catheter is inserted into the artery to open up the vessel and restore the flow of blood. This procedure is called angioplasty. In some cases, a stent, or metal mesh device, may also be inserted to prevent more narrowing in the artery. In hospitals where expert angioplasty is not available within 90 minutes of your arrival, thrombolytic drugs, often called clot busters, are infused into a blood vein in your arm to open the clogged artery. These intravenous drugs dissolve blood clots and usually open the obstructed artery. In most instances, therapy should involve only one of these two options, either angioplasty or thrombolytic drugs. A strategy using both clot-busting drugs and immediate angioplasty may in fact be harmful. Discuss these options carefully with your physician. In most instances, early opening of a blocked artery resolves chest pain quickly, decreases the size of the heart attack, and decreases the incidence of both deadly cardiac rhythm disturbances and heart failure. However, delayed opening of a blood vessel later than 24 hours after a heart attack has begun is no longer worth the risk unless recurrent chest pain or other complications are present.

Q:?? Should I receive blood thinners?

Blood thinners are often used during early treatment of a heart attack to prevent more clots from obstructing the heart's artery. Two groups of blood thinners are prescribed: those that effect platelets and those that interfere with the chemicals that cause blood to clot. Platelets are small, sticky cells that float through our bloodstream to help us clot blood when needed. Anti-platelet drugs cause the platelets to become less sticky. Examples include aspirin and clopidogrel (Plavix). You should be administered 325mg of chewable aspirin as soon as possible following the onset of your symptoms, and clopidogrel should be administered upon arrival to the hospital. Patients already taking aspirin daily should take an additional dose of 75 to 325 mg as soon as possible.

A second group of blood thinners inhibit clot formation by reducing one or more of the chemicals in our blood necessary to form clot. Examples include heparin, enoxaparin (Lovenox), and warfarin (coumadin). Patients in whom fibrinolytic drugs (clot busters) are administered for the treatment of their heart attack are often treated with intravenous blood thinners such as heparin or enoxaparin (Lovenox). These drugs are usually administered for a minimum of 48 hours and often for the duration of the hospitalization, for up to eight days. Heparin should be avoided beyond 48 hours since it may cause blood platelets to dangerously decrease. Warfarin is not used following a heart attack unless complications have occurred such as atrial fibrillation, discussed in a later chapter.

Q:?? Should I be prescribed beta-blockers?

In most instances, beta-blockers are administered early in your hospital course, typically within twenty-four hours. These drugs are discussed in more detail later, but serve to reduce heart rate, promote heart muscle healing, and ward off dangerous cardiac rhythm disturbances. Oral or intravenous beta-blockers should be started within the first 24 hours unless a strong reason exists to avoid them, such as shock, severe asthma, or an abnormally low blood pressure or heart rate. It is also reasonable to administer beta-blockers intravenously upon presentation to the hospital, especially if your heart rate or blood pressure is unusually high.

Q:?? Should I receive angiotensin converting enzyme inhibitors?

This valuable group of heart medicines is discussed in more detail later on, but may be very beneficial if your heart muscle has been badly damaged. This is especially true in the presence of hypertension, diabetes, or chronic kidney disease. Angiotensin converting enzyme inhibitors, or ACEIs, lower blood pressure and help reverse damage to the heart muscle. This is one reason why it is important to know your "ejection fraction." If it is below 40%, you should clearly discuss the use of these drugs with your doctor. Another closely related group of drugs called angiotensin receptor blockers can also be used as an alternative to ACE inhibitors. These drugs may not be prescribed if you have significant kidney trouble, high potassium levels, or unusually low blood pressure.

Q:?? What treatment should I go home on?

If you have been diagnosed with a heart attack and are preparing for discharge home from the hospital, be sure you talk to your doctor about taking the following medications:
- Antiplatelet blood thinners (aspirin and possibly clopidogrel, or Plavix)
- A beta-blocker
- An ACE inhibitor, especially if your ejection fraction is less than 40%
- Nitroglycerine
- Treatment for high cholesterol and high blood pressure as needed

Q:?? How does aspirin help my heart?

Aspirin has a long history in the management of heart disease dating back to Hypocrites in 400 BC. In part, aspirin thins the blood, and reduces the likelihood that a blood clot will form in the heart's arteries. Aspirin is also anti-inflammatory, and helps reduce new areas of plaque formation. Aspirin therefore decreases both the risk and severity of a heart attack and also decreases the chances of developing more hardening of the arteries in the future. Unfortunately, the cardiac benefits of aspirin appear greater in men than in younger women, although older women may benefit somewhat.

Q:?? What's the best dose of aspirin to use?

Despite hundreds of clinical trials, the appropriate dose of aspirin to prevent heart attack and stroke is not entirely apparent. It's clear that one size does not fit all. In men, 81 mg per day consistently lowers the risk of heart attack. In high risk and older women, these doses may not be enough, and 162 to 325 mg daily is often recommended. For stroke prevention, the appropriate dose must be at least 162 mg per day. Since the risk of major bleeding from aspirin at 81 mg per day is the same as it is with 162 mg per day, the most appropriate dose for the primary and secondary prevention of stroke and heart attack is probably 162 mg daily. This equals two low dose aspirins, or half of an adult aspirin. Aspirin should be continued for life after your heart attack. If an angioplasty was performed to treat your heart attack and a stent was placed in the artery, aspirin should be given in a higher dose. For at least one month after placement of a bare metal stent, aspirin (325mg) should be taken. Use 325 mg daily for 3 to 6 months after a drug-eluting stent. Talk to your doctor about what kind of stent was placed during your procedure. After the early phase of recovery, the typical dose of 81 to 162 mg daily can be resumed.

Q:?? Can I stop my clopidogrel (Plavix) after my heart attack?

Clopidogrel works with aspirin to thin the blood. Although their mechanisms of action differ, both drugs work by decreasing the stickiness of platelets. These are small, sticky cells that circulate in the blood stream and are responsible for clotting blood. It's routinely taken in a dose of 75 mg daily. Although clopidogrel may often be prescribed after any heart attack, it is especially important if angioplasty was performed and a stent was placed in your heart. For the first three months following placement of a stent, neither aspirin nor clopidogrel should ever be stopped unless a life-threatening bleeding problem arises. Without clopidogrel, your stent can clot and cause another heart attack. In most instances, clopidogrel should be continued for at least one year, and in some circumstances for as long as two to three years following stent placement. Never allow a physician or dentist to stop your aspirin or Plavix after stent placement without consulting with your cardiologist first. If you are allergic to aspirin, consider clopidogrel as an alternative for lifetime reduction in heart attack risk.

Q:?? Should I have a prescription for nitroglycerine?

All patients discharged from the hospital following a heart attack should be given a prescription for nitroglycerine. Nitroglycerine is available as a small pill or as a liquid sprayed under the tongue. The liquid spray may work slightly faster and has a longer shelf life, although the bottle is slightly larger and deploying the spray may be difficult for patients with advanced arthritis. If chest pain occurs after your return home use nitroglycerine immediately and wait 5 minutes. If the pain is not relieved, a second dose should be taken 5 minutes later. Taking a third dose 5 minutes later is allowed, but is your cue to call 911. Nitroglycerine will do no harm if the chest pain you are experiencing isn't from your heart. Therefore, always error on the side of using nitroglycerine if you are at all concerned about cardiac symptoms. In addition, nitroglycerine can be used to prevent pain. Take it about two or three minutes before an activity that you anticipate may bring about chest discomfort. Nitroglycerine is an unstable product with a short shelf life. It will last longer if kept in a cold, dark location away from fresh air. A good solution is to carry only a few tablets with you, and keep the remaining pills in their bottle in the refrigerator. Every month, replace the few you carry with new tablets.

Q:?? Can I take anti-inflammatory medication?

Many of us need to take medications to treat the aches and pains of getting older! One common group of pain medication used for joint and muscular pain is called "NSAIDS", or non-steroidal anti-inflammatory drugs. Examples include acetaminophen (Tylenol), ibuprofen (Motrin, Advil), and naproxen (Aleve). These drugs may be very helpful, but some may be dangerous for cardiac patients during a heart attack. Ibuprofen (Motrin or Advil) should be discontinued when a heart attack occurs. It increases the risk of hypertension, heart failure, and heart rupture during a heart attack. Ibuprofen (Motrin, Advil) blocks the favorable blood thinning effects of aspirin and promotes salt retention. Therefore, if it is absolutely necessary to use ibuprofen, never take it within two hours of your aspirin. Acetaminophen and additional aspirin are acceptable. If your joints really hurt and don't respond to them, it is reasonable to use a select group of non-steroid anti-inflammatory drugs called nonselective agents. A common example of these agents is naproxen (Aleve), and you should talk to your doctor about other alternatives as well.

Another group of arthritis medicines has created a huge stir recently since they may increase your risk of a heart attack. The selective Cox-2 inhibitors, such as celecoxib (Celebrex), have been associated with an increased cardiovascular risk when used to treat arthritis. This risk appears to be very small but is higher in those with pre-existing heart disease. Therefore, this group of nonsteroidal anti-inflammatory drugs should be considered for pain relief only when intolerable discomfort persists despite attempts at therapy with acetaminophen (Tylenol), aspirin, or naproxen. In all cases, the lowest effective dose should be used for the shortest possible time.

The use of any nonsteroidal anti-inflammatory drug (except acetaminophen) increases the risk of stomach ulcers resulting in a two to four-fold increase in stomach bleeding. Using enteric-coated aspirin may reduce stomach upset but does not reduce the risk of bleeding. If you are at risk of stomach ulcers, talk to your doctor about protecting your stomach against these side effects.

Q:?? Are antioxidants helpful?

The use of antioxidant vitamin therapy to prevent coronary artery disease has been disappointing. For years, supplements such as vitamin E, vitamin C, and beta-carotene were recommended to reduce the risk of coronary artery disease. Since oxidative processes (or rust!) play important roles in the development of arteriosclerosis plaque, antioxidants have been proposed to inhibit plaque formation. At least 15 well controlled studies have evaluated the role of vitamin E, vitamin C, and beta carotene over as long as 12 years to ascertain whether they improve mortality. Collectively, for the most part, clinical trials have failed to demonstrate any beneficial effect of antioxidant supplements on either the severity of illness or mortality from heart disease. In fact, women in one study were given vitamin E plus vitamin C, and had an unexpected increase in their risk of dying. Similarly, an antioxidant cocktail of vitamin E, beta-carotene, vitamin C, and selenium showed more narrowing in blood vessels after 3 years. We suspect that these antioxidants may also interfere with the favorable effects of statin drugs in reducing plaque formation. In a recently reported study of over 14000 physicians followed for ten years, neither vitamin E nor vitamin C reduced the chances of cardiovascular disease. Folic acid and vitamin B have failed to help women or diabetics avoid heart disease in large, lengthy scientific studies. Thus, although we may do well to consume a balanced diet with an emphasis on antioxidant-rich fruits and vegetables, the use of antioxidant supplements is not useful, and may increase risk in some individuals.

Q:?? How about chelation therapy?

Chelation therapy has enjoyed intermittent popularity in the treatment of coronary arteriosclerosis. This treatment involves the intravenous infusions of a medicine called ethylenediaminetetraacetic acid, or EDTA. Claims have been made for years that chelation may rid our arteries of arteriosclerosis. Chelation therapy has now been evaluated in well-controlled scientific studies and is not effective in reducing the risk of heart attack. It is therefore not recommended for the treatment of chronic angina or coronary artery disease, and may be harmful because of the potential to cause low blood calcium levels, allergic reactions, and kidney problems.

Q:?? What treatment occasionally prescribed for heart attacks should I avoid?

Have your doctor discuss with you any of the following treatments prescribed at the time of your discharge. In general, they are prescriptions to avoid unless unusual situations exist:

- Chelation therapy.
- Warfarin for an uncomplicated heart attack.
- Vitamin supplements.
- Anti-oxidant therapy.
- A non-steroidal anti-inflammatory drug.

Controlling risk factors for heart disease

I have followed many patients in my practice for nearly 30 years after their first heart attack. Many still have strong heart muscles, remain employed, and enjoy an active lifestyle. However, it is not possible to enjoy such longevity without significantly modifying the lifestyle that contributes to arteriosclerosis. If you want to live years after your heart attack, you must stop smoking, maintain ideal body weight, exercise regularly, and eat the right food. Arteriolosclerosis is a disease caused by a combination of your heredity and lifestyle. Although we cannot do much about the genes we receive, virtually every risk factor relating to heart disease can be modified and will result in an improved outlook.

Q:?? Is what I eat important?

Eating the right food is essential for you to improve your blood sugar and cholesterol, heal blood vessel inflammation, and improve your overall cardiovascular health. For years, Americans have been eating a diet that is highly processed, rich in calories, and low in nutritional value. We are now paying the price. The traditional western diet destroys the inner walls of our blood vessels, triggers inflammation and clot buildup in our arteries, and promotes blood vessel constriction. Reversing these ravaging effects begins with better food choices. A variety of specific dietary approaches may be tried, but the essentials include:

- Eliminate white carbohydrates (white rice, bread, and potatoes) and favor brown carbs.
- Avoid trans-fats entirely.
- Minimize saturated fats to less than 7% of your total calories.
- Limit total cholesterol to less than 200 mg per day.

The most successful diet for you to accomplish these goals will likely be one that reasonably preserves some of your dietary preferences. So be sure to choose a diet that you will find palatable. For instance, the Mediterranean low carbohydrate diet is quite different from many of the more recently proposed low saturated fat diets, yet accomplishes the same benefits and may be more suitable and therefore successful for some individuals.

Q:?? What about my cholesterol level?

Managing your cholesterol level is absolutely essential following your heart attack. Start dietary therapy immediately upon your return home or even while you're still in the hospital. Reduce your intake of saturated fat to less than 7% of your total calories and reduce your total cholesterol intake to less than 200 mg per day. You should obtain a fasting blood lipid (cholesterol) test soon during your hospitalization for your heart attack. The test measures total cholesterol, the HDL level ("good" cholesterol or "H for happy"), the LDL level ("bad" cholesterol or "L for lousy") and the triglyceride level. Here are your cholesterol targets you should aim for over the next two months:

- Total cholesterol less than 200mg%.
- Triglycerides less than 150mg%.
- HDL level greater than 45mg% in men and 50mg% in women.
- LDL levels less than 70mg%.

If your levels are more than 15% off the target, you will probably require medication to achieve these cholesterol goals, but never give up on your diet. Ask to speak to a dietician in the hospital if you are not well educated about the saturated fat and trans-fatty content of your typical diet. Even if you require medication to lower your cholesterol, the necessary doses will be less if your diet is right!

Lipid-lowering medication is indicated before discharge from the hospital if your LDL is greater than 100 mg%, with a goal of achieving a value of less than 70 mg%. If your triglyceride value is greater than 150 mg% or your HDL is less than 40 mg%, weight reduction and physical activity will be particularly important. If your triglyceride level is greater than 200 mg%, medication is indicated to help reduce your chance of a heart attack as well as protect you from developing inflammation of your pancreas. Niacin and high fiber supplements may help reduce your elevated triglycerides. Lowering your LDL also helps lower the triglycerides as well. The specifics of cholesterol lowering medication are discussed later in another chapter. Supplements such as flaxseed oil and omega-3 fatty acids in the form of fish oil capsules (1 g per day) may also be helpful to you.

Q:?? Am I overweight?

Obesity is becoming a global epidemic in both children and adults. Recent surveys suggest that 66 million Americans are now obese and an additional 74 million are overweight. If these trends continue, one in every five American adults and one in four children will be obese by 2015. Obesity does nothing good. It causes cardiovascular disease, certain cancers, diabetes, stroke, and more absenteeism from work. It also predisposes to lung disease, erectile dysfunction, infertility, sleep apnea, and a higher incidence of surgical complications during operations.

The body mass index, or BMI, measures your "fatness". Figure 4 calculates for you your own BMI by using your body height and weight. In adults, you are overweight if your BMI lies between 25 and 30 kg/meter^2. Obesity is defined as a BMI greater than 30, and morbid obesity as a BMI over 40.

Body Mass Index Table

Height (inches)	Normal						Overweight					Obese										Extreme Obesity															
BMI	19	20	21	22	23	24	25	26	27	28	29	30	31	32	33	34	35	36	37	38	39	40	41	42	43	44	45	46	47	48	49	50	51	52	53	54
	Body Weight (pounds)																																			
58	91	96	100	105	110	115	119	124	129	134	138	143	148	153	158	162	167	172	177	181	186	191	196	201	205	210	215	220	224	229	234	239	244	248	253	258
59	94	99	104	109	114	119	124	128	133	138	143	148	153	158	163	168	173	178	183	188	193	198	203	208	212	217	222	227	232	237	242	247	252	257	262	267
60	97	102	107	112	118	123	128	133	138	143	148	153	158	163	168	174	179	184	189	194	199	204	209	215	220	225	230	235	240	245	250	255	261	266	271	276
61	100	106	111	116	122	127	132	137	143	148	153	158	164	169	174	180	185	190	195	201	206	211	217	222	227	232	238	243	248	254	259	264	269	275	280	285
62	104	109	115	120	126	131	136	142	147	153	158	164	169	175	180	186	191	196	202	207	213	218	224	229	235	240	246	251	256	262	267	273	278	284	289	295
63	107	113	118	124	130	135	141	146	152	158	163	169	175	180	186	191	197	203	208	214	220	225	231	237	242	248	254	259	265	270	278	282	287	293	299	304
64	110	116	122	128	134	140	145	151	157	163	169	174	180	186	192	197	204	209	215	221	227	232	238	244	250	256	262	267	273	279	285	291	296	302	308	314
65	114	120	126	132	138	144	150	156	162	168	174	180	186	192	198	204	210	216	222	228	234	240	246	252	258	264	270	276	282	288	294	300	306	312	318	324
66	118	124	130	136	142	148	155	161	167	173	179	186	192	198	204	210	216	223	229	235	241	247	253	260	266	272	278	284	291	297	303	309	315	322	328	334
67	121	127	134	140	146	153	159	166	172	178	185	191	198	204	211	217	223	230	236	242	249	255	261	268	274	280	287	293	299	306	312	319	325	331	338	344
68	125	131	138	144	151	158	164	171	177	184	190	197	203	210	216	223	230	236	243	249	256	262	269	276	282	289	295	302	308	315	322	328	335	341	348	354
69	128	135	142	149	155	162	169	176	182	189	196	203	209	216	223	230	236	243	250	257	263	270	277	284	291	297	304	311	318	324	331	338	345	351	358	365
70	132	139	146	153	160	167	174	181	188	195	202	209	216	222	229	236	243	250	257	264	271	278	285	292	299	306	313	320	327	334	341	348	355	362	369	376
71	136	143	150	157	165	172	179	186	193	200	208	215	222	229	236	243	250	257	265	272	279	286	293	301	308	315	322	329	338	343	351	358	365	372	379	386
72	140	147	154	162	169	177	184	191	199	206	213	221	228	235	242	250	258	265	272	279	287	294	302	309	316	324	331	338	346	353	361	368	375	383	390	397
73	144	151	159	166	174	182	189	197	204	212	219	227	235	242	250	257	265	272	280	288	295	302	310	318	325	333	340	348	355	363	371	378	386	393	401	408
74	148	155	163	171	179	186	194	202	210	218	225	233	241	249	256	264	272	280	287	295	303	311	319	326	334	342	350	358	365	373	381	389	396	404	412	420
75	152	160	168	176	184	192	200	208	216	224	232	240	248	256	264	272	279	287	295	303	311	319	327	335	343	351	359	367	375	383	391	399	407	415	423	431
76	156	164	172	180	189	197	205	213	221	230	238	246	254	263	271	279	287	295	304	312	320	328	336	344	353	361	369	377	385	394	402	410	418	426	435	443

Source: Adapted from Clinical Guidelines on the Identification, Evaluation, and Treatment of Overweight and Obesity in Adults: The Evidence Report.

Q:?? Why is obesity bad?

Unfortunately, fat tissue is not simply a storehouse for fat; it is really an endocrine organ that is capable of releasing very caustic chemicals into the blood stream that can damage blood vessels. Fatty tissue is also a storehouse for fluid, which may have important repercussions for patients with heart failure. For these reasons, if you are more obese than 85% of the American public, your chances of dying increase by 30%.

As much as obesity is bad, managing your weight will make a big difference. Weight reduction will reduce your heart's size and workload, your blood pressure, arterial resistance, and resting heart rate.

Q:?? How can I lose weight?

Achieving and maintaining a healthy weight throughout life is amazingly difficult in our society. Many factors encourage obesity including large portion sizes, high calorie foods, easy access to inexpensive low nutrient foods, sedentary lifestyle, and commercial and cultural influences that encourage us to eat more calories than we consume.

To reduce weight, use the nutrition fact panel in the ingredient list on the food packages you choose to buy. Eat fresh, frozen, and canned vegetables and fruits without high-calorie sauces. Replace high-calorie foods with fruits and vegetables. Increase your fiber intake by eating beans, all grain products, fruits and vegetables. Use liquid vegetable oils in place of solid fats. Limit your beverages high in added sugar. Cut back on high-calorie bakery products. Select milk and dairy products that are either fat free or low in saturated fat. Use lean meats and remove skin from poultry. Limit processed foods that are high in both saturated fat and salt. Incorporate vegetable based meat substitutes in your favorite recipes.

Here are some tips to help you lose weight. Don't just read them; incorporate each one of them into your daily eating routine as soon as you get home from your heart attack:

- Get rid of white carbohydrates in favor of brown ones (rice, breads, cereals, potatoes).

- A good diet begins in the grocery store. Get bad food out of your house.
- Reduce all of your food portions by 25%.
- Always read every food label carefully.
- Become a member of an organized weight management program.
- Never eat before bedtime.
- Occupy times that you are tempted to snack with physical activity instead.

Q:?? Is eating in restaurants unhealthy?

Americans are consuming more and more food that is prepared outside the home. In the past two decades, consumption of food eaten in restaurants increased from 18 to 32%. Restaurant food is usually larger in portion size, higher in saturated fats and trans-fatty acids, and has higher sugar and sodium (salt) levels. Attaining a healthy diet will require that you make wise choices when you eat food prepared outside the home.

Q:?? Is thyroid disease a cause of heart attack?

Both an overactive and under active thyroid gland can increase the risk of having a heart attack. This is especially true for patients younger than 65 years. Most importantly, the impact that abnormal thyroid function has on heart disease can be controlled by proper treatment. Talk to your doctor to be sure your thyroid function has been measured in the recent past.

Q:?? Does stress play a role in causing a heart attack?

Stress comes in both acute and chronic forms. Examples of acute stress include natural disasters, death in a family member, or the sudden loss of a job. Chronic stress occurs over a long time, and includes marital difficulty and job stress. Both forms are associated with a higher incidence of cardiac events such as sudden, unexpected death and heart attack. It is unclear whether stressful events actually cause hardening of the arteries, or whether they act as triggers for lethal events. Nonetheless, the evidence is overwhelming that proper stress management can both dampen the deleterious effects of stress as well as make us more resilient and less vulnerable to heart attacks. Talk to your doctor about stress management workshops if you feel that stress is having an adverse impact on your happiness.

Q:?? What about depression and heart disease?

Depression commonly accompanies heart disease and actually increases the chances that you will die from it! A mild degree of short-lived depression is acceptable as we face any illness. However, screening for depression and treating it can make a difference in your survival. Talk to your physician about your depression, and don't be fearful of therapy if screening assessments show a problem. In addition, family members should be aware that depression can lead to noncompliance with medication and medical follow-up.

Q:?? I enjoy exercise. Do I need to cut back?

Physical inactivity continues to be a growing problem in our country. Nearly one in four adults report no leisure time activity, while nearly half fail to meet current physical activity recommendations. At the same time, more diseases are being associated with inadequate physical activity. Examples include cardiovascular disease, stroke, hypertension, diabetes, osteoporosis, colon cancer, breast cancer, and depression. All healthy adults need moderate aerobic activity for a minimum of 30 minutes at least five days each week. Your exercise program should stress aerobic forms of exercise such as walking, swimming, or bicycle riding. These activities increase fitness, decrease weight, lower blood pressure, elevate HDL cholesterol and battle depression and stress as well. Low aerobic fitness increases your chances of dying from heart disease, so exercise can prolong your life. However, exercise must be performed wisely. You may wish to talk to your physician about ordering an exercise test to help guide your exercise program. Your exercise sessions can be measured in three ways: frequency, duration, and intensity. Stress frequency (4 to 5 days weekly) and duration (about 30 minutes daily) of exercise, especially early in your program. Intensity is less important. Eventually, you should be encouraged to engage in 30 to 60 minutes of moderately intense aerobic activity such as brisk walking at least 5 days weekly. Resistance training two days of the week may be added. If you absolutely cannot find 30 minutes in the day to exercise, recent data suggests that ten minute sessions performed three times each day may be reasonably equivalent.

You've probably heard of a pedometer, a small device that is worn on your belt to count the number of steps you take each day. Regardless of any particular exercise prescription, patients who wear a pedometer lose more weight and improve their fitness classification. Buy one and use it!

Q:?? Can cardiac rehabilitation help me recover faster?

Definitely enroll into a cardiac rehabilitation program if one is offered near to you. Cardiac rehab is a professionally supervised program designed to help patients recover faster from a heart attack, heart surgery, and cardiac procedures. Most patients who enroll have better compliance with their exercise program, and also have opportunities to be better educated about modifying all of their risk factors. Research has shown us that cardiac rehab participants eat and exercise better, smoke less, have fewer heart attacks, and less frequently require angioplasty and heart surgery.

Q:?? Is coffee a risk for heart attack?

After decades of disagreement and conflicting studies, the relation of drinking coffee and developing coronary heart disease remains unresolved. In most studies, coffee drinking can only be shown to increase the risk of heart attack in smokers, while nonsmokers have little if any increased risk. Nonetheless, if you drink coffee, do so in moderation.

Q:?? What can I do to stop smoking?

More than 46 million Americans are smokers and about 4000 teenagers begin smoking every day. Smoking is an addiction, but stopping is essential to reduce your risk of more heart disease. Smoking cessation will have a greater effect on your health than the effect of any other intervention you can do. Talk to your physician about various ways to stop such as hypnosis or acupuncture. The American Medical Association and American Lung Association websites are a good resource and may be helpful to you. Find times when you feel the need to smoke and fill them with other activities. Try thinking of little tricks to remind you of your challenge to stop smoking. I have one patient who still keeps his last half pack of cigarettes he smoked prior to his heart attack in the sun visor of his truck. Each time he looks at the cigarettes, he remembers the chest pain he had and relives his dedication to stop smoking.

Medication may be helpful as an aide to stop smoking, although be cautious with nicotine gum or patches following a heart attack. Varenicline (Chantix) is a new drug to help smokers stop. It blocks the receptors in the body where nicotine acts and helps reduce craving for nicotine. It also reduces withdrawal symptoms. However, the FDA has recently alerted physicians that users of varenicline may suffer an increased risk of suicide and violent behavior. Drowsiness can also occur that may interfere with driving.

Q:?? What about second-hand smoke?

In addition to active smoking, second hand smoke must also be avoided since it unquestionably increases the risk of heart attack as well as stroke and lung disease. Several researchers have now reported a significant reduction in heart attacks after the introduction of legislation banning smoking in indoor public places. Since heart disease is so prevalent in developed countries, avoiding second hand smoke and banning public smoking has an enormous impact on our risk of disease. When legislation bans public smoking, about two thirds of the benefits are seen in nonsmoking adults! In addition to passive smoking, air pollutants should also be avoided. They raise blood pressure, and promote blood clotting and the progression of arteriosclerosis. Heart attack survivors should carefully assess the healthiness of all of the air we breathe.

Q:?? How vigorously should my diabetes be controlled?

Diabetes is a very important risk factor that increases your chances of having another heart attack or stroke. The prevalence of diabetes is increasing dramatically—about 9% of the adult population now has this disorder. In 2005, one and one-half million new cases of diabetes were diagnosed in people over 20 years of age. In addition to heart disease, diabetes is a leading cause of blindness, kidney disease, and amputation. Uncontrolled diabetes causes damage to the inner lining of the blood vessels and increases their susceptibility to arteriosclerosis.

How tightly diabetes should be controlled has become controversial. Unquestionably, good control reduces the complications of diabetes by at least 10%, and in particular has a favorable effect on reducing kidney disease. However, overly aggressive management may actually increase your chance of dying. Your optimum level of diabetes management should be discussed carefully with your cardiologist and diabetic specialist.

Q:?? Why should I know my hemoglobin A1c value?

We usually think about diabetic control in terms of our blood sugars. A normal fasting blood sugar level is less than 100 mg%. Diabetes is diagnosed when the fasting blood sugar is over 126 mg%. However, blood sugars vary substantially from time to time. The hemoglobin A1c is a blood test that tells you how well your blood sugar has been controlled over the past 3 months. The normal hemoglobin A1c is less than 6.0 mg%. Poorly controlled diabetes causes the hemoglobin A1c to rise. Hemoglobin A1c in excess of 6.5 mg% raises the risk of future heart attack and stroke, and values in excess of eight represent poorly controlled diabetes that dramatically increases your risk. Work with your physician carefully to insure that your diabetic management plan lowers your hemoglobin A1c below 6.5 mg%. If your value continues to be excessive despite the best that you can do, you may want to seek consultation with a diabetic specialist.

Q:?? Should I still receive my vaccinations?

Remember to obtain your annual influenza vaccination. Pneumonia is often preventable, yet accounts for nearly 15% of heart failure cases admitted to our hospitals each year.

How will our lives be changed?

Life should never be the same after a heart attack. Altering the risk factors that contribute to your arteriosclerosis is essential to bail you out of this problem. However, recommendations in the past that markedly restricted patients with heart disease are no longer commonly employed, and most patients should be able to return to a very active lifestyle.

Q:?? What about my sex life?

Yes, you can continue to have wild, hot, sweaty, passionate sex after a heart attack! Actually, sexual activity places a relatively low workload on the heart and can be performed with only a few precautions. Feel open to talk to your doctor about resuming sex after you return home. In most instances, no unusual delays should be necessary. Especially soon after your discharge from the hospital, it is reasonable for you to assume a more passive role, allowing your partner to be more aggressive and active. Keep your overall physical workload at a level that is similar to your walking and general exercise program. Avoid holding your breath or forcibly bearing down. Lastly, remember that your cardiovascular workload is significantly increased when engaging in sex with a new partner so caution is in order!

Q:?? I'm concerned about erectile dysfunction.

For many years, patients have been told that erectile dysfunction (ED) is largely caused by emotional issues. We now know that most cases are caused by diseased blood vessels usually related to arteriosclerosis. As a result, ED not surprisingly occurs in patients who have had strokes or heart attacks. On occasion, ED can be caused by medications used to treat heart disease, especially the beta-blockers. Talk to your doctor about trying alternatives to your medications if ED is a common problem for you.

Q:?? What about Viagra?

Drugs used to treat erectile dysfunction can usually be used by most patients with heart disease. However, they may unfavorably interact with long-acting forms of nitroglycerin. If you occasionally use tadalafil (Cialis), vardenafil (Levitra), or sildenafil (Viagra), make sure to always include them on your medication list. When these drugs are taken in conjunction with nitroglycerine, severe low blood pressure can occur and may be very difficult to treat. Nitroglycerine in a pill or capsule form should be avoided for 24 hours after using sildenafil or vardenafil, and for 48 hours following the use of tadalafil. Since intravenous nitroglycerine is often used when you come to the hospital complaining of chest pain, be completely honest with hospital personnel and remind them if you have recently used these drugs.

Q:?? When can I return to work?

Most patients can plan to return to their previous employment following recovery from their heart attack. Specific guidelines are very difficult to discuss since many factors impact on whether and when you should return to work. This matter should be discussed with your doctor prior to your discharge from the hospital. In discussing your eligibility to return to work, you need to know how severely your heart attack impaired your heart function. You also need to know how prone you are to another heart attack. Your physician needs to know what kind of work you do and how much physical labor is involved. You may get back to work earlier if your work schedule and duties are flexible or if you can return to work on a part-time basis. Many patients with a small to moderate uncomplicated heart attack can return to work in two to three weeks. Larger, more complicated heart attacks may preclude work for six to eight weeks.

Q:?? I'm elderly. Are there any special concerns with my heart attack?

Symptoms of a heart attack in the elderly may be somewhat different than in younger individuals. Chest pain tends to be less severe and more commonly completely absent, while shortness of breath and fatigue are more common. According to current studies, older persons respond as well to treatment for a heart attack as do younger people. Specifically, their response to angioplasty, beta blockers, ACE inhibitors, and cholesterol-lowering drugs are quite similar. The elderly are less frequently candidates for thrombolytic, or clot busting, drugs due to concerns about bleeding complications.

Q:?? What about using female hormone replacement therapy?

A confusing array of conflicting information is available to women regarding estrogen replacement therapy. Over the years, the doses of estrogen and progestin replacement have changed, and the quality of the studies to follow their impact has varied. Current guidelines conclude that hormone therapy with estrogen and progestin, or estrogen alone, should not be given to postmenopausal women with the intention of preventing future heart attacks. Postmenopausal women who are already taking estrogen plus progestin, or estrogen alone, at the time of a heart attack should discontinue hormone therapy. In the hospital, hormone therapy should not be continued while you're at bed rest due to an increased risk of blood clotting. Women who have been taking hormone therapy for at least one to two years and who want to continue treatment because of postmenopausal symptoms need to recognize a small increased risk of cardiovascular events and breast cancer with combination therapy as well as stroke with estrogen therapy.

Q:?? What about cocaine use?

The widespread use of cocaine and methamphetamines make it important to consider these drugs as potential causes of a heart attack. Cocaine can cause the heart arteries to spasm and obstruct. They also can cause the blood to clot more easily, promoting a heart attack in people who have existing blockages. If cocaine has been used and chest pain occurs, nitroglycerin should be used immediately to relax the blood vessel and prevent a heart attack from occurring. If nitroglycerin is not effective, oral calcium blockers such as diltiazem (Cardizem) or nifedipine (Adalate, Procardia) may be helpful. Most importantly, be certain to confide in your doctor and list all of the drugs you have been taking prior to your heart attack, including illicit drugs. The management of your heart attack may be different if you're honest.

Q:?? What's new about cocoa?

Flavanols are chemicals contained within certain plants and are found plentifully in dark chocolate, red wines, black tea, and cocoa. Flavanols may decrease the incidence of heart attacks by improving the overall health of our blood vessels and make them less susceptible to arteriosclerosis. They may also lower blood pressure.

Q:?? What life style changes are a must?

Before you go home from the hospital, know what lifestyle changes you will need to make, and have a plan for each one. Specifically, you need to know:

- How you will lose weight.
- How to exercise wisely.
- How to stop smoking.
- What foods to eat and what to avoid.
- How you can enroll in a cardiac rehab program.
- How to manage stress.
- The optimal management for your diabetes.
- What medication you will be taking when you go home.
- When is your follow-up appointment with your doctor.

I Have Heart Failure

Q:?? What is heart failure?

Heart failure, also called congestive heart failure or CHF, sounds like a complex term but is really quite simple. Heart failure means that the heart muscle is too weak to pump enough blood to meet the body's needs. The bloodstream delivers all of the nourishment to the body and carries away the waste products to the kidneys for removal. When the heart becomes weak, every organ suffers from mal-nourishment, and poisons accumulate. The kidneys are particularly sensitive to decreased blood flow, and kidney impairment during heart failure is common. The term "congestive" describes the tendency for excessive fluid that cannot be excreted from the body to flood organs and interfere with their function.

The major symptoms of heart failure are shortness of breath, swelling, weight gain, and fatigue. Shortness of breath results from fluids flooding the lungs. Excessive fluid during the day when we are upright usually gravitates down into our legs causing swelling or edema. A good way to detect retained fluid is to press your shinbone with one finger for three to four seconds. Withdrawing your finger should not leave an indentation that you can feel. If it does, suspect swelling. When we lie down at night, gravity may gradually pull the fluid from our legs to our lungs, resulting in shortness of breath that awakens us from sleep. Patients with heart failure often find sleeping upright on several pillows or in a chair more comfortable than lying down flat.

Q:?? How can I prevent heart failure?

Heart failure is a relapsing disease, and you will need to approach it with long-term management in mind. The hallmark of early heart failure is water retention. This is usually evident by swelling in the feet, increasing shortness of breath, or more than a 2-pound weight gain on any one day. It is important to weigh yourself the first thing every morning, on the same scales, and before you put your clothes on. Generally, an increase in weight of two pounds or more reflects fluid retention. Talk to your doctor about allowing you to change your daily diuretic (water pill) dose when you detect water retention. In most patients, the same dose of a diuretic every day just doesn't work. The dose needs to be changed since the amount of fluid you retain varies from time to time. I often give patients what's called a "sliding scale" of diuretic doses. This technique is really quite simple. Your usual dose of diuretic, say 40mg of furosemide, is taken when you are at your dry weight, perhaps 182 – 184 pounds. If your weight increases to 185 – 186 pounds, your dose should increase to perhaps 80 mg. If your weight increases above 186 pounds, your dose may increase to 120 mg, or a second diuretic may be added. Similarly, if you become somewhat dry and your weight slips below 182 pounds, your diuretic dose will be reduced or perhaps eliminated. These changes in your medicine doses need to be customized to your own situation, but work with your doctor to see if you can play a more proactive role in the management of your heart failure.

Q:?? Is salt restriction important?

Restricting salt in your daily diet is important in the management of heart failure. Salt intake promotes water retention. Don't forget about the high levels of salt commonly found in restaurants and processed foods. Actually, your diuretics will work better with some salt in your diet, so that excessive salt restriction is usually unnecessary. For most patients, a total of 2300 milliequivalents of sodium (or salt) each day will be enough to avoid trouble. You will need to read food labels regularly and become aware of salty foods if you want to achieve this target. Avoidance of salty foods usually suffices with no added salt at the table. Excessive water intake should also be avoided. It is unnecessary for most patients to force fluids or try to drink extra water every day. Drink enough water to answer your body's thirst.

Q:?? How should my heart failure be evaluated?

Two questions need to be answered to manage your heart failure. The first is why you have heart failure, and the second is what brings it on. Any form of heart disease may lead to heart failure. For example, an old heart attack or a badly functioning heart valve may result in enough damage to the heart muscle to cause heart failure. It is important for you to know the cause of your heart failure, since in some cases treating the cause reduces the risk of recurrence. As an example, improving the heart's blood supply through surgery or angioplasty or fixing a defective heart valve may strengthen the muscle enough to avoid failure.

In addition to evaluating the cause for heart failure, the factors that trigger a particular episode need to be investigated. The most common trigger of heart failure is failing to take your medication properly. Excess salt or water intake may also be a culprit. Other common causes include febrile illnesses, lung conditions, or sudden arrhythmias of the heart. In most instances, the cause of heart failure can be discovered following an honest discussion with your doctor. In more perplexing cases, additional testing may be necessary to understand what has aggravated your heart condition.

Q:?? What treatment should I receive?

The first tactic in the treatment of heart failure is to appreciate the underlying cause, and be as aggressive as possible in fixing it. Thus, patients with heart failure due to blockages in blood vessels may respond well to angioplasty or surgery in an effort to improve blood supply to the heart muscle. Heart failure due to a leaky valve may require valve replacement or repair.

Lifestyle changes are essential. You must optimize your body weight, stop smoking, and using caution regarding salt and water intake. Recent evidence confirms that patients who exercise regularly reduce their risk of heart failure. However, you need to establish carefully chosen exercise guidelines with your physician as excessive exercise may be risky.

Medication is essential to prevent heart failure. Four groups of medications are useful and all may be necessary. Angiotensin-converting enzyme inhibitors, or ACE inhibitors, are medications that reduce salt and water retention, and dilate blood vessels to make it easier for the heart to pump blood. Many ACE inhibitors are now available and are discussed in more detail later in this book. Beta-blockers slow down the heart rate and reduce the high adrenaline levels often seen during heart failure. A diuretic, or water pill, is crucial in most cases to keep excessive fluid from overloading the heart. Lastly, spironolactone is a special kind of diuretic that also reduces the heart's workload and may improve its function. Adjusting doses of these medicines is important to avoid low blood pressure, low heart rate, and to avoid adverse effects on kidney function or electrolyte levels in the body. Therefore, you should work carefully with your physician especially during the early phases of treatment to be sure these medicines are used carefully. A home blood pressure cuff can be very helpful to understand adverse effects to your medications. A digital machine using an arm cuff is usually sufficient and reasonably accurate, and blood pressures taken once or twice per day during the early phases of treatment may help your physician determine your tolerance to these medications.

Q:?? What medication should I take for heart failure?

In summary, ask your physician if you are taking the following medication to treat your heart failure:

- An ACE inhibitor or angiotensin blocking agent.
- A diuretic or water pill.
- Spironolactone.
- A beta blocker.

Q:?? What medication should I avoid?

If you have heart failure and take any of the following medication, talk to your doctor about why they've been prescribed and whether it is wise for you to continue them:

- Salt retaining drugs such as arthritis medication and alka seltzer.
- Calcium channel blockers.
- Digoxin.

Q:?? How will living with heart failure change my life?

Heart failure can almost always be treated and a great deal can be done to prevent the illness. As your body's excess fluid is eliminated, the heart becomes smaller in size and develops stronger contractions. Hormones produced during heart failure that promote salt and water retention diminish. Thus, heart failure waxes and wanes. Proper diet, regular exercise, losing excess weight, and taking your medications faithfully are vital strategies to minimize your chances of having heart failure. Never be embarrassed to go over your medication list carefully and repeatedly until you are sure you understand each medication. Learn to manage your own heart failure with your physician. Monitoring your daily water intake, checking your daily weights and changing your diuretic dose according to your weight and amount of swelling is a very effective means of keeping you away from the hospital. This will mean that you will have to create a trusting and interactive relationship with your physician. However, the goal is to keep you well and at home.

No one can learn to understand and treat your heart failure as carefully as you can.

Q:?? Why do heart failure patients return to the hospital so frequently?

Patients hospitalized for heart failure have a higher likelihood of going back into the hospital within 30 days of discharge than any other diagnosis in medicine. You can help avoid this problem by working with your physician to help manage fluid retention. You need to learn how to alter your medication doses to manage your own body fluid levels. You need to know about the salt content of the food you eat, and be conscientious about avoiding it. You must take your medication faithfully, and be sure to schedule a follow-up appointment with your physician within a few days after discharge.

I Have Atrial Fibrillation

Disorders of the regular rhythmic beating of the heart are called arrhythmias. The most common of these is atrial fibrillation. About 2.2 million Americans live in atrial fibrillation. Nearly one in twenty five of us will experience this arrhythmia in our lifetime.

Q:?? What is atrial fibrillation?

The upper chambers of the heart are called atria and are composed of millions of muscle cells. In a normal heartbeat, all of the cells contract together. However, things don't always go as planned. In fibrillation, the electrical activity in the upper chambers becomes completely chaotic, and every heart cell contracts on its own. The result is like a symphony without music, with each instrument playing its own song. The organized contraction in the upper chamber is lost and replaced by a chaotic quivering of the heart muscle. This is called atrial fibrillation.

Atrial fibrillation results in two problems. The first problem is an abnormally fast and irregular heartbeat that can be quite uncomfortable for many people. The normal heart rate is responsive to circulating hormones and nervous system messages. For instance, if we are sleeping the sinus node stimulates the heart with perhaps 50 or 60 impulses each minute. As we exert or become emotionally excited, the impulses increase in frequency and our heart rate speeds up. In atrial fibrillation, the sinus node can no longer control the heart rate, and our hearts speed up even when we're quiet and inactive. For many patients, atrial fibrillation results in complaints of irregular palpitations, fatigue during exertion, and shortness of breath due to the unrestrained rapid rate.

The second problem caused by atrial fibrillation is blood clotting. Blood circulating in our bodies wants to clot whenever blood flow stagnates. When contraction in the upper chamber ceases, the flow of blood slows and clots can form. These clots may break away from the heart and travel to distant places. A clot flowing to the brain is a leading cause of stroke.

Q:?? Does atrial fibrillation have different forms?

You may hear your doctor say that atrial fibrillation occurs in different patterns. We speak of paroxysmal atrial fibrillation that comes and goes over time. Persistent atrial fibrillation begins and does not stop until treatment is begun. Chronic atrial fibrillation never ends despite all available treatment. Within five years of the first episode of paroxysmal fibrillation, about 25% of patients will progress to the chronic form. This more commonly occurs in elderly patients and those with significant underlying heart disease. Patients who do not have heart disease will more likely have paroxysmal episodes.

Q:?? What causes atrial fibrillation?

In most instances, some form of heart disease causes atrial fibrillation. Examples include prior heart attacks, leaky or narrowed heart valves, cardiomyopathy or weakness of the heart muscle, or an overactive thyroid gland. We usually order tests to evaluate for these conditions, including an electrocardiogram, echocardiogram, and blood tests for thyroid function. Don't forget to ask your doctor about blood tests for thyroid function, since hyperthyroidism, or overactive thyroid function, may produce atrial fibrillation as its only symptom. This is especially true in older individuals. In addition, it represents a curable form of atrial fibrillation. About 20% of those with atrial fibrillation have nothing wrong with their heart that produces it. These patients are said to have "lone" atrial fibrillation.

Q:?? What triggers atrial fibrillation?

Even after many episodes of atrial fibrillation, most patients cannot identify any factors in their life that seem to trigger a particular episode. However, some patients do find that what they eat or drink, or how well they exercise or sleep, may trigger a particular event. Alcohol ingestion may be a factor for some patients. Over the counter cold medicines containing pseudoephedrine (e.g. Sudafed), caffeine, and sleep deprivation may trigger episodes. Occasionally, patients may predictably arise with atrial fibrillation in the early morning hours, a pattern referred to as "cholinergic atrial fibrillation." Keep track of your episodes and the events in your life surrounding them to see if any pattern evolves. If so, this may help your physician choose more specific therapy to ward off further occurrences.

Q:?? How is atrial fibrillation treated?

We have two different approaches in our treatment of atrial fibrillation. In the first approach, we allow atrial fibrillation to persist, but control the heart rate with medication and lifestyle changes. This strategy is often called "rate control," and is designed to minimize symptoms from fibrillation. Calcium channel blockers (diltiazem, verapamil) and beta blockers (metoprolol, atenolol, propranalol, nadolol) are frequently prescribed for this purpose. Although digoxin (Digitek, Lanoxin) is also prescribed to control the heart rate, recent evidence suggests that it may be detrimental to your health and should probably be avoided in most instances. You should discuss rate control with your doctor especially if you tolerate atrial fibrillation and the medications necessary to control the rate, or have had atrial fibrillation for a long time, making it unlikely that a normal rhythm can be restored.

The second strategy is called "rhythm control," which attempts to suppress atrial fibrillation and maintain the normal rhythm of the heart. In contrast to a rate control strategy, you may prefer rhythm control if you tolerate atrial fibrillation poorly, have side effects to the medications necessary to control heart rate, or have developed atrial fibrillation recently. Examples of medications to prevent atrial fibrillation include propafenone, sotalol, dofetilide, and flecainide. You may wish to stay clear of amiodarone, since most patients who have atrial fibrillation will be prone to recurrent episodes for many years. Although amiodarone can be used safely for the short-term management of atrial fibrillation, this drug is associated with numerous long-term toxic side effects, and its long-term use should be discouraged. A few new drugs will soon be available, so stay tuned with your doctor to evaluate newer options.

Q:?? What is ablation?

In addition to medication, a procedure called ablation may be useful to prevent episodes of atrial fibrillation. Several forms of ablation can be performed. In some instances, we can eliminate atrial fibrillation by performing an ablation. For example, in some patients atrial fibrillation arises in the pulmonary veins, or those tubes that drain the blood from the lungs back to the heart. This is particularly true in young people who do not have heart disease. A small catheter is placed into these veins, and thermal energy is used to ablate, or eliminate the areas where atrial fibrillation originates. Thermal energy can also be used to create linear channels in the upper chambers. This process organizes the electrons as they flow through the atria, eliminating the chaotic flow of electrons. Many ablation procedures utilize combinations of these techniques. When considering ablation, you need to speak in detail with your physician about the potential success rates and complications. Serious complications occur in 2-5%, and success rates are generally reported to vary from 70 to 90%. Thus, at least one in ten patients will not have a successful procedure, and as many as one in twenty may have a serious complication. These facts need to be weighed seriously in your decision to proceed with ablation. Nevertheless, ablation is the only cure for atrial fibrillation and may be a good option for you to avoid years of heart medication and concern about blood clot formation.

A different and simpler form of ablation is called atrioventricular nodal (or AV node) ablation. In this procedure, a permanent pacemaker is inserted before the ablation. The electrical connection between the upper and lower chambers of the heart is then destroyed using a heat-tipped catheter. This is a far simpler procedure, and virtually uniformly successful. After AV node ablation, your heart rate will be regular, and the rate will be determined by the setting of your permanent pacemaker. Therefore, most patients who have AV node ablation will no longer sense the presence of atrial fibrillation and no longer require medication to control the rate. However, it is important to understand that your atria will remain in fibrillation, and the risk of blood clots will still be present. Therefore, anticoagulants (blood thinners) may still be necessary. In addition, your own heart rate without your pacemaker will be very slow, and you will essentially become dependent upon your pacemaker. Although pacemakers are extremely reliable from a technical standpoint, you should speak with your doctor about the concept of pacemaker dependency and what this may mean to you. In most cases, catheter ablation of the AV node should not be attempted without a prior trial of medication to control the arrhythmia.

Q:?? Should I take anticoagulants?

Most of my patients do not like taking blood thinners. Anticoagulants, or blood thinners, require frequent blood tests to dose them properly. Minor bleeding is a constant complaint, and the fear of major bleeding is always looming. Nevertheless, atrial fibrillation is responsible for about 15% of strokes, and blood thinners are our only proven protection. Fortunately, not all patients with atrial fibrillation require blood thinners. We recognize six important risk factors that predispose to blood clots. These include poor heart muscle function, diabetes mellitus, hypertension, valve disease, advancing age particularly over 75 years, and a history of a prior stroke. If none of these risk factors are present, the likelihood of a blood clot is less than 1% per year, and the risk of taking warfarin cannot be justified. In such patients, aspirin (81 mg in males and 162 mg in females) is recommended. If two or more risk factors are present, the risk of a clot climbs to between five and ten percent each year, and the risk of taking warfarin is clearly justified. Even though bleeding complications do occur with warfarin in about 1- 2% of patients per year, bleeding is usually less hazardous to you than the risk of stroke. If you have one or more of the risk factors for clot formation, speak with your physician about your risks of stroke and compare them to the risks of bleeding on warfarin. Individual decisions are important, since the use of warfarin always represents a decision based on the balance between the risk and benefit of the drug.

Clopidogrel (Plavix) is not indicated in the treatment of atrial fibrillation. The risk of bleeding is about the same with clopidogrel and warfarin. However, clopidogrel has very little if any benefit in reducing clot formation when used for atrial fibrillation.

Warfarin (Coumadin) is the standard drug for patients who need blood thinners. Warfarin works by depleting the amount of vitamin K in the body, a critical building block for blood clotting substances. To measure the blood thinning effect of warfarin, a blood test is performed called an international normalized ratio, or INR. The higher the INR, the thinner the blood. A normal INR is less than 1.5. A target INR of 2-3 is adequate for most patients with atrial fibrillation. An INR below 2 does not protect against blood clot, and an INR higher than 3 results in more bleeding with no additional protection. An INR should be determined at least weekly during initiation of therapy until your INR level reaches a stable and desirable level. If you have atrial flutter, which is a close cousin to atrial fibrillation, the same blood thinning therapy is recommended. Warfarin cannot be given during the first trimester or last month of pregnancy, and an intravenous blood thinner called heparin, should be substituted.

One more comment about atrial fibrillation. The guidelines that dictate the need for blood thinners to prevent strokes have been well circulated amongst physicians since the middle or end of the 1990s. Nevertheless, warfarin remains amongst the most under-prescribed medications relative to the guidelines that require its use. If you have or have had atrial fibrillation in the past, be sure to discuss fully with your doctor whether blood thinners are indicated for you.

Q:?? How will atrial fibrillation affect my future?

Most patients who have atrial fibrillation can lead a normal life, although medication will be necessary to control fibrillation and thin the blood. Patients who are highly symptomatic impress me when atrial fibrillation first begins, but adapt quickly to it and in short time can no longer tell they're in fibrillation.

I have high blood pressure

Q:?? What is normal blood pressure

Everybody requires a blood pressure. Without it, blood cannot circulate through our bodies. Two numbers are recorded when measuring your blood pressure. The top number is called the systolic pressure and measures the pressure in your arteries generated by each heartbeat. The bottom number, called the diastolic pressure, measures the persisting pressure in the arteries while your heart rests between beats.

Many years ago, the normal systolic blood pressure was thought to be 120mm Hg plus your age. This ridiculously high value was abandoned years ago, and the arbitrary level of 140/90 was selected as the upper limits of normal. We now know that the risk of heart attack and stroke continues to decline as blood pressure drops. This is true even within the normal range of pressures. Therefore, the risk of a heart attack is lower with a blood pressure of 110/60 than one of 138/88. Our present treatment goal is to reduce blood pressure to an average of 115/75 (120/80 during daytime and 100/65 during the night), while avoiding side effects from pressures that are too low, such as weakness and lightheadedness.

Q:?? Why is high blood pressure important?

Hypertension afflicts up to 27% of adult Americans. It is a common and important risk factor for stroke, heart attack, and kidney failure. The complications of high blood pressure increase as your average daily blood pressure increases. Slowly on, the inner walls of the blood vessels become stiff and less elastic, and are more prone to hardening of the arteries. Over longer periods, the kidneys lose their ability to filter blood, the heart becomes thickened and subject to arteriosclerosis, and the brain develops arteriosclerosis and hemorrhage. It is unfortunate that high blood pressure causes no symptoms until a catastrophic problem occurs. This disease has clearly earned its reputation as the silent killer of many Americans.

Q:?? Why do I suddenly have high blood pressure?

The kidneys are the cause of most high blood pressure. They have two distinctly different jobs. One is to cleanse the blood of poisonous chemicals made during normal body metabolism, and excrete them in the urine. The second function is to read the blood pressure and excrete an enzyme called angiotensin into the blood stream to regulate it. When the blood pressure is too low, the kidneys excrete more angiotensin. This retains salt and water and constricts blood vessels. By doing so, the pressure in the system increases. In contrast, if blood pressure is too high, angiotensin secretion decreases. This relaxes blood vessels and eliminates salt and water from the body. As a result of these actions, blood pressure decreases. In most individuals, hypertension is caused by an abnormal amount of angiotensin excreted from the kidneys.

Several risk factors increase the likelihood of having high blood pressure. Treatable risk factors include a body mass index of 30 or higher (being overweight), excess salt intake, lack of physical activity, and excessive alcohol ingestion. Other risk factors for hypertension that cannot be as easily controlled include race, heredity, and advancing age.

Q:?? Is it important to monitor blood pressure at home?

Blood pressure is measured by a sphygmomanometer, one of the oldest tools in cardiology. Home digital models are now available that are easy to use and reasonably priced. An arm cuff is more accurate than a wrist cuff, and finger cuffs should be avoided. A home cuff gives you the advantage of measuring your blood pressure at different times of the day, since some individuals will have high pressures only in the morning or evening. The readings can also be obtained more frequently and under more quiet circumstances than in a doctor's office, reducing the chance of the "white coat syndrome." However, don't forget to bring your cuff in with you to the doctor's office about once a year to verify that it is working correctly.

Q:?? Does treating high blood pressure decrease my risk?

Fortunately, high blood pressure is almost uniformly treatable. Even small reductions in blood pressure can have enormously beneficial effects. A 3mm reduction in systolic blood pressure results in 8% fewer strokes and 5% fewer heart attacks. Lowering systolic blood pressure by 20mm Hg reduces cardiovascular risk in half. The "20/10" rule states that for every 20/10mmHg decrease in blood pressure, cardiovascular mortality risk is cut in half. Thus, the cardiovascular risk for a patient whose blood pressure is 115/75 is half that of a patient whose blood pressure is 135/85.

Q:?? How is high blood pressure treated?

The cornerstone of hypertension management is to modify the lifestyle factors associated with it. Regular exercise, weight management, reduction in alcohol intake, and restriction in dietary salt are essential. These measures often are sufficient to treat mild hypertension, and will reduce the amount of medication required to control more severe cases. Weight directly correlates with blood pressure, and numerous studies have documented that weight loss lowers blood pressure. Modest weight loss can reduce blood pressure by 20% among those who are overweight.

In addition to weight management, proper diet is important to prevent and treat hypertension. On average, as dietary salt (or sodium) intake increases, so does blood pressure. Recent recommendations suggest that an ideal salt intake should be limited to 1500 mg per day to ensure adequate nutrient intake. In the Western diet, this may be very difficult to achieve, and a reasonable recommendation is to restrict the upper limit of sodium intake to 2300 mg per day. To do this, choose foods low in salt and do not add salt at the table. Since over 75% of consumed salt comes from processed foods, evaluate food labels carefully and buy wisely.

High potassium intake reduces blood pressure, especially in African Americans. To increase your potassium intake, consume foods rich in potassium such as fruits and vegetables. It is reasonable to attempt to increase your potassium intake to 4700 mg per day. This is far in excess of the average intake of potassium in our country of 2900 to 3200 mg per day. These recommendations apply only if you have normal kidney function. If your kidney function is abnormal, speak to your physician about whether your dietary potassium can be supplemented.

Q:?? Can I still drink alcohol?

Recent studies have documented a direct, dose-dependent relationship between your alcohol intake and your blood pressure, especially if you drink more than two drinks per day. An alcoholic drink is usually defined as 12 ounces of beer, 5 ounces of wine, or 1.5 ounces of 80 proof distilled spirits. Alcohol consumption should be limited to two or fewer drinks per day for most men and one or fewer drinks per day in women or lighter weight men.

Q:?? What medications are available to treat high blood pressure?

Medication to treat hypertension is important when lifestyle factors are insufficient to control blood pressure. Numerous well-controlled clinical trials have now concluded that reducing your blood pressure reduces your chance of stroke, heart attack, and kidney failure. The main classes of medications used to treat hypertension include diuretics, beta-blockers, calcium channel blockers, angiotensin-converting enzyme inhibitors, and angiotensin receptor blockers.

Diuretics (or water pills) are often the first drugs prescribed for early hypertension. You can think of managing high blood pressure in the same way as changing the water pressure in the plumbing system of your house. If you remove a few gallons of water from the pipes in your house, turning on the faucet would reveal a significant reduction in water pressure. Similarly, blood pressure will go down if diuretics reduce your body's fluid volume. Hydrochlorothiazide is the principal diuretic prescribed for hypertension. Some patients treated with diuretics require potassium pills since diuretics also wash potassium from the body. In most instances, you should ask for a blood test to check your potassium value shortly after a diuretic is prescribed. Diuretics in common use include hydrochlorothiazide (Hydrodiuril, Esidrix, Microzide), indapamide (Lozol), bumetanide (Bumex), furosemide (Lasix), spironolactone (Aldactone), and chlorthalidone (Hygroton). Some people suffer from attacks of gout after prolonged treatment with diuretics. If you are diabetic, ask your doctor about the effect that diuretic drugs may have on diabetes. Changes in your diabetic medication or diet may be necessary.

Beta-blockers are a common group of drugs used to treat hypertension. These drugs block the part of the nervous system that is responsible for increasing our heart's rate and force of contraction. Examples include propranolol (Inderal), metoprolol (Lopressor; Toprol), nadolol (Corgard), atenolol (Tenormin), bisoprolol (Ziac, Zebeta), acebutolol (Sectral), betaxolol (Kerlone), pindolol (Visken), timolol (Blocadren), and carvedilol (Coreg). Side effects to beta-blockers include fatigue, tiredness, and sexual dysfunction, particularly in men. Less common side effects include insomnia, cold hands and feet, or worsening of asthma. If you take insulin for diabetes, be aware that symptoms from low blood sugar may be much less pronounced when taking beta-blockers. If you take allergy shots, be sure your allergist knows that you are taking a beta-blocker.

Calcium channel blockers are also used to treat high blood pressure. The middle layer of the blood vessels of our body is composed of muscle. Calcium moves through small channels in the muscle causing the muscle to contract. Calcium channel blockers relax the muscles of our arteries by inhibiting the movement of calcium. In this sense, taking channel blockers is like replacing the one inch pipes in your plumbing system with more elastic two inch pipes. When the water is turned on, the pressure will be lower. Examples of calcium channel blockers include verapamil (Calan, Covera, Isoptin, Verelan), diltiazem (Cardizem, Tiazac), nisoldipine (Sular), felodipine (Plendil), isradipine (DynaCirc), nicardipine (Cardene), nifedipine (Adalat, Procardia), and amlodipine (Norvasc, Lotrel). In general, calcium channel blockers are well tolerated and do not lower potassium or adversely effect kidney function. They may cause constipation and may occasionally reduce heart rate. Swollen ankles may occasionally result, especially from amlodipine.

Angiotensin is an enzyme in the kidney that is at the root of hypertension, and a chemical in our kidneys called angiotensin converting enzyme (or ACE) is responsible for its formation. Since producing lots of ACE leads to high blood pressure, inhibiting the secretion of ACE or blocking its activity will lower blood pressure. Angiotensin-converting enzyme inhibitors include lisinopril (Zestril, Prinivil), ramipril (Altace), enalapril (Vasotec), monexipril (Univasc), trandolapril (Mavik) perindopril (Aceon), quinapril (Accupril), benazepril (Lotensin), and captopril (Capoten). These agents may occasionally raise potassium levels or adversely affect kidney function. Therefore, you should remind your physician that blood tests for potassium and kidney function may be important shortly after beginning an ACE inhibitor. Some patients may also become allergic to ACE inhibitors over time. This may result in a skin rash, swelling in the throat or lips, or a dry, annoying cough. When this occurs, angiotensin blocking agents are often substituted for ACE inhibitors. These drugs accomplish the same reduction in angiotensin activity, but do so by blocking the receptor where they work rather than decreasing angiotensin formation. They may be used alone or in combination with ACE inhibitors. Examples include candesartan (Atacand), eprosartan (Teveten), irbesartan (Avapro), lasartan (Cozaar), telmisartan (Micardis), and valsartan (Diovan). Angiotensin receptor blockers cause side effects similar to ACE inhibitors, but do not usually cause the chronic dry hacking cough seen with ACE inhibitors.

Some of the drugs now used to lower blood pressure are combination products using two drugs from different groups. For example, Zestoretic is a combination between lisinopril and hydrochlorothizide, and Lotrel is a combination between amlodipine and benazepril. Combination products have the advantage of taking one pill each day rather than two, and may reduce your costs somewhat if both medicines are necessary. However, talk to your doctor about delaying the use of combination products until after the best dosages for each drug have been determined.

No single treatment is the best answer for all patients. A compelling reason to select a certain drug may exist if your hypertension is associated with other diseases. For instance, if you have hypertension as well as coronary artery disease, an ACE inhibitor or beta-blocker may be the best choice. In diabetes, ACE inhibitors may be useful since they also help protect the kidney against the injurious effects of diabetic kidney disease. When hypertension is associated with heart failure, an ACE inhibitor or angiotensin receptor blocker, with or without a beta-blocker, may be useful.

Q:?? How do I take my medication?

Blood pressure varies considerably during a normal day. It is lower at night and exhibits a steep increase in the early morning. Heart attacks and strokes are more likely to occur during this vulnerable early morning time, so that taking medication at night, or if necessary taking it twice daily, may further reduce your risk. Irregardless, taking blood pressure medicine for some people is harder to remember because high blood pressure causes few symptoms. Therefore, get in the habit of taking medicine at a time when it is easy for you to remember and develop a habit of taking it the same time each day.

Q:?? How will my life change with high blood pressure?

Hypertension is a disease that often causes no symptoms despite dangerously high blood pressure levels. Therefore, the life of a hypertensive patient may not be affected despite the presence of uncontrolled hypertension until a complicating stroke, kidney failure, or heart attack occurs. It is therefore extremely important to regularly monitor your blood pressure. Most patients can monitor the effects of their own treatment by purchasing a home blood pressure cuff. Arm cuffs are more accurate than wrist or finger cuffs, and a digital system is reliable and reasonably inexpensive. Home blood pressure monitoring allows you to obtain more blood pressures at different times of day, and in an environment that is familiar to you. Keep a log of your blood pressure, and don't hesitate to bring it in to talk to your doctor. Home monitors are especially important for the elderly who cannot leave their home easily, pregnant women, and those with kidney disease whose blood pressure may vary frequently over large ranges. Taking readings at home will also encourage you to cut your risks: use less salt, exercise more, and lose weight. Be aware that high blood pressure usually causes no symptoms, so that staying on your medicine despite feeling well is very important. High blood pressure treatment will be necessary for the rest of your life. Do not stop treatment when your blood pressure improves.

Adhering to lifestyle changes that favorably affect blood pressure is crucial. Remember that while high blood pressure is usually treatable, treatment can be complicated and must be individualized. Don't be discouraged if several prescription trials are necessary to find the right treatment for you. Always remember that the inconvenience of long-term medication is still better than living with a stroke or a heart attack.

I have high cholesterol

Q:?? Why is cholesterol important?

High cholesterol is a leading cause of hardening of the arteries, or arteriosclerosis. This disease affects the blood vessels of the neck and brain leading to stroke, and the heart's blood vessels leading to myocardial infarction or heart attack. How cholesterol damages the inner lining of our blood vessels is still being intensively studied. Damage begins with inflammation in the inner lining of the blood vessels causing small microscopic cracks. The body repairs these cracks by deploying cells through the blood stream that dive into the cracks and plug the holes. Unfortunately, LDL cholesterol, the main building block of repair cells, is left behind in the crack resulting in plaque build up. Both inflammation and high cholesterol are required to produce plaque, and lowering your cholesterol levels clearly improves the health of your arteries.

Q:?? What can I do to lower my cholesterol?

Making healthy food and lifestyle choices is essential to lower your cholesterol. Maintaining an ideal body weight is the first step. In general, females should consume no more than 1600 to 2200 calories per day, while males should have no more than 2400 to 2800 calories per day to maintain ideal weight. For most of us, a conscious decision is necessary at mealtime to lower our proportions and achieve these calorie restrictions. In addition to the quantity of food, the quality of our food is also important. Eat foods that are nutrient rich but low in calories. Replace high-calorie foods with fruits and vegetables. Concentrate on eating deeply colored vegetables and fruits such as spinach, carrots, peaches, and berries. Eat whole vegetables and fruits instead of drinking juices that often have added sugar and salt. Use liquid vegetable oils and soft margarine in place of hard margarine and shortening. Limit cookies, crackers, and French-fries made of partially hydrogenated or saturated fat. Read the ingredients list before you buy your food. Pay special attention to serving size to understand how much fat and cholesterol you are really eating. Keep your total cholesterol intake to less than 200 mg/day. If you drink alcohol, drink in moderation, limiting yourself to one drink per day for women and smaller men, and two drinks per day for larger men. If you have a sweet tooth, eat dark chocolate in moderation. It dilates your coronary arteries and decreases clot formation. This action may relate to bioflavonoid epicatechin activity in the chocolate.

Three blood fats need to be lowered, including total cholesterol, LDL (or "bad") cholesterol, and triglycerides. Unfortunately, our genes strongly influence these values making it necessary for some individuals to watch their diet extremely carefully. Total cholesterol and LDL cholesterol are lowered by a low-fat, high fiber diet. Triglycerides also correlate positively with the occurrence of arteriosclerosis, and should be lowered along with total cholesterol. Triglycerides respond more to our total caloric intake and our activity levels, and correlate closely with obesity.

Q:?? When is cholesterol too high?

Obtain a cholesterol panel at least annually and more often if you are trying to correct elevated values. Know your numbers and compare them to the following tables to assess your risk of heart attack and stroke:

Blood Value	Risk
Total Cholesterol	
<200mg%	Optimal
200-239 mg%	Borderline to high risk
>240 mg%	High risk

HDL Cholesterol (remember "H" for happy):

>50 mg%	Optimal
<40 mg%	High risk (men)
<50 mg%	High risk (women)

LDL Cholesterol (remember "L" for lousy):

< 100 mg%	Optimal
100-129mg%	near optimal

130-159mg%   borderline high

160-189mg%   high

Triglycerides:

<150 mg%   Optimal

150-199mg%   Borderline high

200-499mg%   High

>500 mg%   Very high

The goals of the American Heart Association are to have you lower your total cholesterol below 200 mg%, and raise HDL cholesterol to above 45 mg% in men and 50 mg% in women. Triglycerides should be lowered below 150 mg%. LDL cholesterol should be lowered below 130 mg% in everyone, and below 100 mg% in higher risk individuals with diabetes, hypertension, or who have a family history of arteriosclerosis at an early age. For those who have already had a heart attack or stroke, LDL should be lowered to 70 mg%. Lowering your LDL level has an amazing impact on your risk of disease. The incidence of stroke and heart attack can be reduced by 2% for every one point decrease in LDL. This means that reducing your LDL from 150 mg% to 120 mg% may lower your risk by 60%!

HDL cholesterol is also related to your stroke and heart attack risk, but inversely so. This means that low HDL raises your risk and a high HDL protects you. Raising the HDL cholesterol may be particularly important since HDL mediates reverse cholesterol transport, a process that is responsible for reversing hardening of the arteries. HDL cholesterol also has anti-inflammatory and antioxidant effects that may further help keep you healthy. Your HDL cholesterol needs to be elevated above 45 mg% in men and 50 mg% in women. While the risk of a major cardiovascular event increases by nearly 25% for every 5 mg% drop in HDL, a 1% increase in HDL corresponds to a nearly 3% reduction in your risk. To raise your HDL level you must exercise regularly, maintain an ideal body weight, use low to moderate doses of alcohol, and consider treatment with niacin. Niacin, or nicotinic acid, is a form of vitamin B3. It is the drug of choice for increasing

HDL levels, helping to drive cholesterol out of the fatty plaques. Some patients find niacin unacceptable because of skin flushing. If you suffer from this side effect, begin at a very low dose (250mg daily) and slowly increase the dose over several weeks. In some patients, the use of a long-acting form of niacin may minimize side effects, although the impact on HDL may be slightly blunted. Aspirin may lessen this side effect if taken about one to two hours before your niacin.

Q:?? What about high cholesterol medications?

In many individuals, our rigorous goals for LDL and total cholesterol reduction are unachievable by diet and exercise alone. In most circumstances, a good diet will be successful in lowering cholesterol by perhaps 15%. Cholesterol levels above 250 mg% or an LDL value exceeding 150mg% may present a challenge to you that cannot be accomplished by diet alone. If this is the case, medication may be needed. In many individuals, reductions in total cholesterol of 50-100%, and reductions in LDL cholesterol of 75- 100% are achievable by medication.

Statin drugs are the most common medications used to reduce total cholesterol and LDL cholesterol. These powerful drugs prohibit cholesterol production in our livers and drastically reduce cholesterol blood levels. Statins may possibly be the single biggest contributor to the reductions in heart attacks and strokes that we have witnessed over the past decade. Examples of statin drugs include atorvastatin (Lipitor), fluvastatin (Lescol), lovastatin (Mevacor), pravastatin (Pravachol), rosuvastatin (Crestor), and simvastatin (Zocor). All of these statins have been shown in well controlled scientific studies to reduce the incidence of both primary and secondary heart attacks and strokes. These drugs cannot be used in pregnant or breast feeding women or in women of childbearing age. They should be used cautiously in patients with liver disease.

Q:?? Are the side effects to statin drugs worth it?

Statin drugs have side effects, as do all drugs. Muscular inflammation is the most common complaint. About 3 to 5% of patients complain about muscle soreness usually within the first four months of therapy. Patients who are frail and thin or have low thyroid function are at highest risk. Most patients describe an aching sensation sometimes associated with tenderness to touch. On occasion, actual muscular weakness may occur. The muscle pain may be continuous or intermittent, but usually persists until the statin is stopped. The pain is clearly in the muscles rather than in the joints where arthritis hits. Symptoms usually improve if you stop the drug for one or two weeks. In very rare cases, intense muscle inflammation has resulted in the release of chemicals from the muscle cells that damages the kidneys and can cause death.

Unfortunately, many patients remain reluctant to use statin drugs because of these reported side effects. We are all concerned about side effects to medication, and want to avoid damage to our bodies. Comparing statins to the use of seatbelts in your car will help you understand why statin drugs are a good choice for you. Very few of us would feel comfortable driving without a seatbelt since we know they markedly reduce our risk of injuries. However, we also know that injuries may rarely be caused by a seatbelt. Since we don't know in advance what will happen to us in a car accident, we use a seatbelt and take our chances. Using a statin drug follows the same logic. Side effects can occur and can rarely be very dangerous or even fatal. However, the risk of a stroke and heart attack is markedly reduced with these medications, and on balance our probability of living a long life will increase. Many studies enrolling thousands of patients randomized to take either a statin drug or a placebo (an inactive pill), have shown that despite exposure to side effects, statin drugs save lives. More people live longer with statins than without them.

A few tricks may be helpful to you if muscle inflammation is troublesome. Talk to your doctor about trying fluvastatin (Lescol), which has the lowest risk of muscle toxicity. Also, alternate-day therapy or even weekly therapy has been promoted to help avoid this side effect. An interaction may be present between statin drugs and amiodarone (a rhythm controlling drug) that may increase the incidence of muscle inflammation.

Statin drugs may also rarely cause problems with liver function, and blood tests for liver function should be done once or twice yearly. If only minor elevations are noted, it is not always necessary to stop the statin. Many of these test abnormalities become normal in time even if you continue the medication. If the liver tests do not improve, a smaller dose may be used. In some instances, the drug must be stopped to allow liver enzymes to normalize, and an alternative statin may be tried at a future time.

Q:?? I can't tolerate statins. Are there alternatives?

Alternatives to statin drugs do exist to treat your high cholesterol. Bile acid binding drugs are active in your intestines. They bind fat and inhibit its absorption into your body. Examples include cholestyramine (Questran, LoCholest) and colestipol (Colestid). Bile acid binding drugs can decrease your chances of a heart attack. The drugs are safe although gastrointestinal distress and constipation may occasionally occur. If you use these drugs, increase your water intake to help with the constipation. Also be aware that these drugs may interfere with the absorption of other medication, such as thyroid replacement hormones, diuretics, and blood thinners like warfarin. Ezetimibe is a newer drug that inhibits the absorption of cholesterol. It is well tolerated, rarely causes muscle inflammation, and can often be used in combination with a statin drug. For example, Vytorin is a combination of simvastatin and ezetimibe. One recent inconclusive study suggested that lowering your LDL with ezetimibe may not be as effective as a similar reduction with simvastatin.

Q:?? How can I increase my HDL?

Drugs can also help increase your HDL cholesterol level. Examples include niacin, fenofibrate (Antara, TriCor), and gemfibrozil (Lopid). Niacin can be quite effective in raising the HDL as well as lowering the LDL. Be aware that "dietary supplements" of niacin may actually contain a highly variable amount of niacin (sometimes none at all!). Use caution in combining gemfibrozil with a statin drug, as the incidence of muscle inflammation may be considerably increased. If you choose to use a fibrate in combination with a statin, fenofibrate may be a better alternative.

Q:?? What about lowering triglycerides?

Omega-3 fatty acids taken as "fish oil capsules" in doses of 3 to 4 g per day are frequently used to lower triglycerides. These substances can be found naturally in oily, cold water fish such as salmon and lake trout, as well as many dark green leafy vegetables. Studies have shown that fatty acids may reduce triglycerides, lower blood pressure, and produce mild blood thinning. However, some studies suggest that patients who have heart failure or markedly weakened heart muscles should not take fish oil, since it may increase the risk of sudden death.

Q:?? What is recommended for children with high cholesterol?

Due to the high incidence of heart disease in our society, children should have their cholesterol measured every 3-5 years beginning at age two. Nutritional therapy should begin in the first year of life if members of the child's family are obese or have heart disease. The same fat restrictions and exercise programs we use for adults should be instituted in children. In youngsters who persist with high cholesterol, drug therapy should now be considered at eight years of age.

I have cardiomyopathy

Q:?? What is cardiomyopathy?

Cardiomyopathy is a disease of the heart muscle. The term "cardio" refers to your heart. The term "myopathy" means heart muscle weakness. We categorize cardiomyopathy into three types. Dilated cardiomyopathy is the most common variety and results in an enlarged, weakened heart. Hypertrophic cardiomyopathy is the second type. "Hypertrophic" means that the heart muscle is thicker and stiffer than normal. The third form of cardiomyopathy is called restrictive cardiomyopathy and is quite rare. In this form, the heart muscle is infiltrated with foreign substances that make the heart stiff and resistant to filling with blood.

Dilated cardiomyopathy may often follow a viral infection of the heart. In most cases, dilated cardiomyopathy presents slowly with insidious progression of shortness of breath and fatigue. It less commonly has an acute presentation called acute myocarditis. Patients with myocarditis become suddenly ill and complain of severe weakness, sudden severe shortness of breath and fever. Dilated cardiomyopathy is a very serious condition, although the prognosis has improved dramatically in recent years, and many patients may improve substantially or even achieve total remission from their disease. A few causes of cardiomyopathy are treatable, such as those caused by drugs or excessive alcohol abuse. When being evaluated for dilated cardiomyopathy, it is important to be honest with your physician about all the medications, drugs, and alcohol that you have taken in the past.

Q:?? What is broken-heart syndrome?

Researchers have recently reported a new form of dilated cardiomyopathy formally called Takotsubo cardiomyopathy. What a name! This syndrome is often seen after a serious emotional event, and is more commonly given the name "broken heart syndrome." The disease causes severe heart muscle weakness and heart failure. It may be caused by high levels of circulating adrenaline during the time of an extremely severe stress. Almost all patients with this disorder regain normal heart muscle function within a few weeks.

Q:?? What is hypertrophic cardiomyopathy?

Hypertrophic cardiomyopathy results from an unusual thickening of the heart muscle. A hypertrophic heart looks like a body builder on steroids! Causes include severe untreated hypertension, stenosis or narrowing of the aortic valve, and an inherited condition that occurs in families. It is much more common in males. Hypertrophic cardiomyopathy may not produce any symptoms until the disease is advanced. It causes dangerous rhythm disturbances, and is a leading cause of sudden unexpected death in young athletes. Hypertrophic cardiomyopathy should be suspected in young male patients who complain of significant palpitations, shortness of breath on exertion, or who show findings on physical examination or electrocardiogram of increased thickness of their heart muscle. Be particularly suspicious if you have a family history of sudden unexpected cardiac death in young people.

Q:?? What is restrictive cardiomyopathy?

Restrictive cardiomyopathy is a rare diagnosis. In this disorder, the heart muscle becomes stiffened and cannot expand and dilate to receive incoming blood. This is usually due to infiltration of the heart muscle by foreign substances like iron or amyloid. In most circumstances, restrictive cardiomyopathy is a complication of other diseases that affect the whole body.

Q:?? How is cardiomyopathy evaluated?

The most useful test to evaluate patients suspected of having a cardiomyopathy is the echocardiogram. This test is explained in more detail later, but is basically an ultrasound test used to define the structure of the heart and how well it functions. In dilated cardiomyopathy, an enlarged heart is seen with thin walls and a weak contraction. In hypertrophic cardiomyopathy, the walls of the heart are thickened and extra strong, and the contraction of the heart is overly vigorous. In restrictive cardiomyopathy, the heart muscles are thickened and unusually dense. Contraction force may be preserved.

The electrocardiogram may also be helpful in evaluating cardiomyopathy. Although the EKG cannot specifically diagnose cardiomyopathy, it is useful as a screening tool especially in adolescent athletes during a routine pre-season physical examination.

Q:?? How is cardiomyopathy treated?

Each form of cardiomyopathy is treated differently. Patients with dilated cardiomyopathies are treated similarly to those with heart failure. Angiotensin converting enzyme (ACE) inhibitors or receptor blockers and beta blockers form the basis of treatment. As dilated cardiomyopathy weakens the heart, the body releases large quantities of a chemical called angiogtensin to increase the amount of blood pumped by the heart. This chemical has very deleterious effects, including blood vessel constriction and salt and water retention that hasten cell death. The result is a vicious cycle that further weakens the heart and produces yet more angiotensin. Angiotensin enzyme inhibitors and receptor blockers interfere with this vicious cycle by inhibiting the action of angiotensin. Beta blockers help decrease the heart rate, which promotes heart recovery and reduces the workload on the heart. Spironolactone may also be helpful and may be added in many cases. Blood pressure and heart rate should be kept in the low to normal range. In advanced cases, implanted defibrillators may be useful to help prolong survival. In summary, if you have a dilated cardiomyopathy, talk to your doctor about receiving the following treatment:

- A beta blocker.
- An angiotensin converting enzyme (ACE) inhibitor or receptor blocker (ARB).
- A diuretic.
- Spironolactone.
- Consideration for an implanted defibrillator.

In hypertrophic cardiomyopathy, beta-blockers are the treatment of choice. These drugs restore more normal heart contraction and decrease the heart's vulnerability to abnormal and dangerous rhythm disturbances. As in dilated cardiomyopathies, defibrillators may be useful in selected patients who are at high risk for sudden death. Vigorous physical activity may need to be restricted.

Restrictive cardiomyopathy presents an enormous therapeutic challenge. Very little has been developed to help the prognosis in this disease. In some instances, the underlying systemic disorder that infiltrates the heart muscle may be treatable or at least modifiable. As the blood builds up behind the heart waiting to enter its stiffened cavity, diuretics (water pills) may be useful to improve symptoms.

If your cardiomyopathy does not respond to treatment, consideration should be given to cardiac transplantation. Transplant medicine has improved enormously in the last decade, giving added years and better functional capacity to many patients. Availability of hearts for transplant continues to be the limiting factor. If your cardiomyopathy does not improve within the first six months of treatment, or symptoms continue to significantly impair your activity despite the best available treatment, begin to talk to your doctor sooner rather than later about cardiac transplantation.

Q:?? How will cardiomyopathy change my life?

Cardiomyopathy is a chronic disease that will require you and your doctor to work together to improve your long-term outlook. Medications have significantly improved the prognosis for most patients. Compliance with your medication and lifestyle changes are equally important. Restricting salt and optimizing your body weight will ease the burden on your heart and help it heal. Some restriction in activity may be required, especially in the hypertrophic form of cardiomyopathy. Your participation in competitive sports should be discussed at length with your doctor. However, regular exercise at moderate workloads remains extremely important to improve your fitness, decrease the workload on your heart and help optimize your weight.

Remember also that some forms of cardiomyopathy, particularly of the hypertrophic type, are heritable. Your siblings and your children may require echocardiograms or EKGs to determine whether they have also been afflicted with the disease. Blood tests are now available commercially to identify the genes responsible for the inherited forms of this disease, and should be considered to better define your cardiomyopathy and its prognosis, as well as to identify the disease in your offspring.

Chapter 3: Diagnostic Tests for My Heart

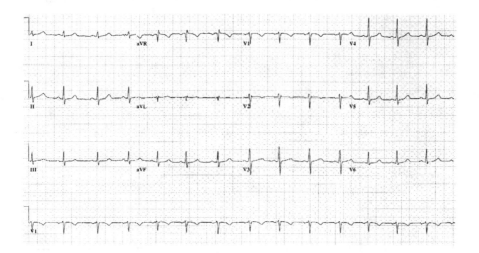

The electrocardiogram

The electrocardiogram, abbreviated as an EKG or ECG, was one of the first tests developed to assess heart disease. It is a painless test with no side effects. The EKG involves the placement of small stickers on the skin over the legs, arms, and across the front surface of the chest wall that measure the electrical activity of each heartbeat. While gazing at a statue in a museum, you would likely want to view it from multiple angles. In this way, we get a better appreciation for what the statue really looks like. Similarly, the electrocardiogram views the electrical impulses as they go through the heart muscle from 12 different angles. Therefore, it is often referred to as a 12-lead EKG. Figure 5 shows an example of a normal EKG:

Each normal heartbeat results in three blips, or waves, recorded as deflections over time. The first small defection is called a P wave. The P wave results from contraction of the upper chambers (atria). The second larger deflection is referred to as the QRS complex. The QRS complex results from contraction of the lower chambers of the heart. The last of the deflections is called the T-wave. The T-wave represents electrical relaxation of the heart's lower chambers.

The electrocardiogram still remains a very useful test for evaluation of heart disease. It also the main test we use to diagnose the heart's rhythm. The normal rhythm of the heart results from an electrical discharge from the sinus node that causes the upper chambers to first contract followed by the lower chambers. As such, it is referred to as a normal sinus rhythm. Many abnormalities may replace normal sinus rhythm, and are discussed throughout this book. Examples include atrial fibrillation and heart block. These abnormalities are easily identified on an EKG. The electrocardiogram can also be used to diagnose enlargement of the chambers of the heart, damage to the heart muscle from new or old heart attacks, as well as diseases of the pericardium, or outer lining of the heart.

A few limitations in the use of EKGs are worth mentioning. An EKG may be entirely normal in patients with chest pain who are about to have a heart attack, and therefore cannot be used to completely reassure you that pain in your chest is not of concern. An old heart attack may no longer appear on an EKG. We can therefore not confidently reassure people that they have not had a heart attack in the past by an EKG. Lastly, most cardiac rhythm abnormalities come and go. The EKG will be normal if it is performed at a time that your arrhythmia is not present.

The echocardiogram

The echocardiogram, or cardiac ultrasound, is commonly used to evaluate the anatomy and function of the heart. In this test, high frequency sound waves are sent from the front of the chest wall down to the heart. The process is similar to the way a submarine uses sonar to find its way around the ocean. As the sound waves encounter the heart muscle and valves, they reflect back to the chest wall. The echo machine then creates an image of all four chambers of the heart and its valves. Doppler technology is often performed with the echocardiogram to study the rate of blood flow through the heart and the pressures of blood generated by the heartbeat.

The echocardiogram is a painless test and has no risk. If required, the echocardiogram can be repeated frequently. On occasion, a fair amount of pressure is necessary while applying the transducer to the chest wall that may result in mild discomfort.

Cardiac stress testing

Exercise testing is used to detect blockages in the blood vessels that supply the heart with blood. Exercise is usually performed on a treadmill, although a bicycle can also be used. As you exercise, the speed and incline of the treadmill will increase every 3 minutes. Generally, the test is continued until you no longer desire to exercise. Optimally, at least 85% of your maximum obtainable heart rate should be achieved for good diagnostic accuracy. During the test, your heart rate, heart rhythm, electrocardiogram, and blood pressure should be monitored regularly. Some form of imaging of the heart may be added to the study to improve its accuracy. For instance, a radioactive material may be injected into the bloodstream that flows to the heart muscle. The radioactive material cannot flow to an area of the heart if the blood supply is blocked. Therefore, images looking for blockages will show the absence of radioactive activity. Ultrasound, or echo, imaging of the heart is an alternative to radioactive studies. If the blood supply is blocked, the heart muscle may become weaker with exercise rather than stronger as we usually see. Each of these tests has relative advantages and disadvantages, and neither is perfect in detecting heart problems. Talk to your doctor before your test to understand which test is best for you.

Cardiac stress testing is a safe test, although some risk of complications does occur during maximal exercise. Overall, the complication rate should be well under one in 1000 tests. A physician trained in cardiopulmonary resuscitation and exercise testing should be available at all times during the test, and emergency resuscitation equipment should be available in the event of complications.

Q:?? Can blockages always be detected by exercise testing?

The accuracy of exercise testing depends on several issues. First, the stress posed on the heart must be fairly high. At least 85% of your highest heart rate during exercise should be achieved. Your maximum heart rate can be determined in several ways, but the simplest is to subtract your age from 220 beats per minute. Using this formula, the maximum heart rate during exercise for a 65 year old would be 220 – 65, or 155 beats per minute. Be sure to talk to your doctor before your test if you are concerned about any ailments that may restrict your ability to fully exercise. Secondly, your routine electrocardiogram should be relatively normal in order for changes during exercise to be appreciated and understood. If your electrocardiogram prior to testing is not normal, the addition of some form of imaging of the heart to supplement the electrocardiogram during exercise will be important. Lastly, your medications may influence the results of your test. Talk to your doctor before your test to determine whether any medication you take may adversely effect the results.

With these limitations in mind, an exercise study will accurately detect blockages in about 85% of patients with significantly obstructed arteries. This means that up to 15% of patients may have a normal exercise test despite threatening disease. In other words, an exercise test is a helpful guide, but the results should not be used to completely exclude blockages in your arteries, especially if you have worrisome symptoms or significant risk factors that predispose you to coronary artery disease.

Also be aware of false positive responses to exercise testing. This means that an exercise test may be abnormal in some cases in the absence of any heart disease. Although a false positive response is not common, an exercise study should never be considered diagnostic of coronary artery disease, especially in patients at low risk.

Recording cardiac rhythm

Sporadic rhythm changes of the heart are hard to diagnose. An electrocardiogram only records brief moments of the heart's rhythm and is usually not being performed while symptoms are present. Therefore, an EKG often misses the diagnosis. Longer sampling of cardiac rhythm is possible by using 24 hour or one-month recording systems. In a 24-hour recorder, often referred to as a Holter recorder, electrodes are applied to the front wall of the chest using adhesive patches. A recording box carried on your belt for 24 hours continuously records cardiac rhythm. Try to be normally active during your test. Many cardiac rhythm disturbances may relate to activity, and being inactive hides them. If your cardiac symptoms are infrequent, you may want to discuss the possibility of a month-long recording device with your physician. These devices are often referred to as event recorders. This device works somewhat differently than a 24 hour monitor, in that the device saves examples of abnormal rhythm detected by the device software and also records rhythm when told to by the patient. A small button on the device can be pushed at any time that you are having symptoms. Each time that you push the button, remember to enter the symptoms you are experiencing in a diary. For patients with very infrequent symptoms, a small recording device called a loop memory recorder can be implanted under the skin below the left collarbone. This small microchip can either be triggered to record rhythm by a small button carried with you, and can record rhythm changes on its own. These devices are particularly useful for patients who have palpitations or fainting spells that occur very infrequently.

Cardiac catheterization

Cardiac catheterization is a test to evaluate for valve problems and blockages in the coronary arteries. Small tubes are placed in the arteries and veins of the body, usually in the groin area. These tubes then slide up the arteries and veins toward the heart. The blood pressure and flow rates in the heart are measured to determine how well the heart muscle and the heart valves work. Pictures of the heart muscle are taken to confirm how well it contracts. Most importantly, contrast material, sometimes called dye, is injected through the tubes into the blood vessels of the heart. In this way, blockages can be detected and measured.

Q:?? What are the risks of cardiac catheterization?

Cardiac catheterization is a diagnostic test that carries some risk. Bleeding or infection can occur where the catheters are placed. The contrast material, or dye, that is injected to take pictures of the blood vessels may cause allergic reactions. More severe anaphylactic reactions with shock can rarely occur. If you have ever received an injection of contrast material in the past, it is very important to share with your physician any adverse affects you may have experienced. The kidneys can also fail after exposure to contrast material. Kidney damage most commonly occurs in patients with pre-existing kidney disease and in diabetics. Medication can be given to you prior to your catheterization to reduce the chances of allergic reactions and kidney damage. It is very important to talk with your physician before your catheterization to assess ways that will make your catheterization safer. Examples include proper hydration, proper monitoring of blood thinners, pre-medication to prevent allergies and kidney damage, and awareness of other blockages in blood vessels such as the carotid arteries or aorta.

All physicians who perform catheterization report a very small incidence of complications. However, complications correlate closely to the number of catheterizations a physician has performed. Don't be hesitant to ask your physician about his experience with this procedure. You may wish to entertain a second opinion if your physician performs fewer than 50 cardiac catheterizations per year, especially if he is a younger physician newer to the practice of invasive cardiology.

Q:?? What recommendations do I follow after my catheterization?

A catheterization is usually performed through an artery in the groin. Following your procedure, you will need to remain reasonably inactive for a few hours in order to prevent any bleeding from the site. Although you can be up and about, walk slowly and take care going up or down steps. It is normal to have slight discomfort at the site of the catheterization, but you should not experience severe, throbbing pain. Black and blue discoloration of the skin commonly occurs and may extend several inches below the groin site, especially in the few days after the catheterization. However, a bulging beneath the skin that feels like a tennis ball or orange is not normal and should be reported to your physician.

CT Angiography

A CT angiogram, or CTA, is a new test designed to view the coronary arteries without catheterization. Phenomenal increases in computer speed now make it possible to actually see the coronary arteries and determine whether blockages are present using CT (or CAT) scans. The test often requires oral or intravenous medication to slow the heart rate before the procedure. Contrast material, or dye, is injected through an intravenous line. Within seconds of the injection, the coronary arteries can be seen in their entirety. CTA is proving extremely accurate to confirm that you have normal coronary arteries. However, if blockages are present, CTA may fall short in defining their severity. "Soft plaque" is a term used when little if any calcium is contained in a blockage. CTA is more accurate in identifying the extent of narrowing when soft plaque clogs an artery. However, CTA may not be as accurate when "hard plaque" is present that contains high levels of calcium. In these cases, cardiac catheterization may still be necessary to address the severity of narrowing.

Several limitations and complications of CTA should be kept in mind. Approximately the same amount of injected contrast material used in catheterization is also required for CTA. Issues about contrast allergies and kidney damage still apply. Some experts are also concerned about the long-term risk of cancer that may result from the high levels of radiation used during CTA. You should discuss these side effects carefully with your cardiologist before your procedure to determine whether you have sufficient probability of disease to warrant the risks of CTA. Use CTA prudently!

Chapter 4: Treatment for heart disease

I need a pacemaker

Q:?? What does the heart's electrical system do?

Electrical impulses in the heart cause the heart muscle to contract. This jolt arises from the sinus node, located in a small area in the upper right chamber. Think of the sinus node like a spark plug. Many times every minute, the sinus node sends out a small electrical spark to the rest of the heart. As we exercise, the sinus node speeds up its rate of electrical stimulation. As we sleep, the rate of stimulation decreases. Each small spark that the sinus node makes travels through wires to the upper chambers, causing the muscle to contract. After the upper chambers contract, the electricity converges on a small structure joining the upper and lower chambers called the atrioventricular (or AV) node. From the AV node, electricity conducts through more wires called bundle branches down to the heart's lower chambers, where a second contraction results. Thus, the normal sequence of the heartbeat is an upper chambered contraction followed slightly later by a lower chambered contraction.

Q:?? Why do I need a pacemaker?

Defects in the normal function of the electrical system can occur at any location in the heart. The sinus node may malfunction, depriving the heart of needed electrical stimuli. When seriously malfunctioning, the sinus node may actually stop for short periods, resulting in an absent heartbeat with fainting. The wires, called bundle branches, that conduct electricity from the sinus node to the heart muscle may also become defective. This condition is called heart block or bundle branch block, and occurs to varying degrees.

A pacemaker is often required when the heart's electrical system fails. Pacemakers are electronic devices designed to replace a faulty electrical system. The purpose of a pacemaker is to provide the heart with an electrical stimulus from a battery. Most pacemakers are "demand" pacemakers since they work only when needed. Demand pacemakers can sense when a normal heartbeat exceeds a set rate, and do not compete. When the heartbeat slows below a certain rate, the pacemaker turns back on and stimulates the heartbeat. In this way, a demand pacemaker works like your home's thermostat, turning on the furnace only when needed.

Q:?? How is a pacemaker inserted?

A pacemaker is composed of two parts. A small metal can measuring about 1-1 ½ inches in diameter and ¼ inch thick contains the pacemaker's computer parts and battery. This is called the pacemaker generator. It is placed through a small incision just below the collarbone under the skin. Below the collarbone lies a blood vein, through which small wires, called leads, thread down to the heart. In most implants, one lead is placed in the right lower chamber and one in the right upper chamber. On occasion, only one lead is required to either the upper or lower chamber. A small screw on the end of the lead fixes it to the inner lining of the heart muscle. The other end of the lead is then attached to the pacemaker generator. The generator is placed under the skin below the collarbone and the incision is sutured closed.

Q:?? How long will the pacemaker's batteries last?

Pacemaker batteries usually last about seven to eight years. At some point during the follow-up of your pacemaker, testing will show that the battery voltage is getting low. Don't panic! You will need to be scheduled in the near future to have the pacemaker generator changed. The skin over the pacemaker will need to be opened and the generator replaced with a new one. The entire generator that you feel under the skin will be changed, not just the battery. This ensures that you will have the latest in technology available in your new unit. In most instances, the old leads will still be functioning normally, and can simply be re-connected to the new generator. On occasion, the leads may also show defects and new leads may be required.

Q:?? What complications can occur during a pacemaker insertion?

A pacemaker insertion usually causes mild discomfort around the incision for three or four days. Three common complications can occur during or after an implant. Infection is a risk with all incisions, and usually requires that the entire pacemaker and wiring system be removed so that the infection can heal. Below the blood vein used to advance the leads to the heart lies the lung, which can be nicked as the wires are advanced to the heart. A small tube must then be placed between the ribs to evacuate air and allow healing to occur. Lastly, leads may dislodge from their original position in the heart because of the heart's constant beating. This may not pose a risk to you, but the incision will need to be reopened and the leads moved to a different location. Rare complications include perforation of the heart muscle and bleeding. Hiccups can rarely be noticed following implantation of a pacemaker due to stimulation of the breathing diaphragm by the pacemaker's electrical stimuli. All in all, complications of pacemaker implantation should not exceed 1-2%.

Q:?? What should I know before going home with my pacemaker?

Before going home from the hospital, you should receive a temporary card that lists the name of your pacemaker's manufacturer, the model number of your pacemaker and leads, and a toll-free number to call the manufacturer if you should have any questions about your pacemaker. In a few weeks, you will be mailed a permanent card. The computer that is used to communicate with a pacemaker is different for each manufacturer. It is very important to keep your pacemaker identification card with you when you travel so that caregivers anywhere will know the manufacturer of your device. If you are in a remote part of the country and having problems that you suspect may be due to your pacemaker, you can also use the toll-free number on your card to find a physician familiar with your pacemaker who practices near you.

Some restrictions in your activities may be necessary for a few days. You should be sure that moving your shoulder and arm is comfortable before you resume driving. Most patients should refrain from driving for at least 4-7 days. You will want to ask about restrictions in activities such as golf, bowling, or carrying heavy items. Be sure your physician knows what kind of physical activity is required during your work before asking when you may return to your job. You may be asked not to lift the arm on the side of your pacemaker above your head for a few weeks to reduce the chances that the leads will come loose. Be sure to have an appointment with the physician responsible for your pacemaker's follow-up before going home.

Q:?? How will having a pacemaker change my life?

A pacemaker should not significantly restrict your lifestyle. A brief outpatient pacemaker test will be required about two to four times each year. During these evaluations, a computer mouse is placed over your pacemaker. This test ensures that the pacemaker's circuit boards and leads are working correctly, and also estimates the remaining battery life. In about 7 or 8 years after your implant, the test will show that the pacemaker's battery is beginning to deplete. Your follow-up tests are extremely important, and you should be sure each time you are finished with your exam that your next evaluation is scheduled.

Q:?? Are any precautions needed because of my pacemaker?

We all know that our environment is filled with invisible electronic signals coming from many sources such as cell phones, pagers, televisions and radio transmitters. Day to day, few precautions are required to be sure that none of the signals interfere with your pacemaker. It is safe to be around most household electrical equipment such as cordless phones, household appliances, electric blankets, ipods, hair dryers, and office equipment. It is reasonable to keep household power tools and radio transmitters at least 12 inches away from your pacemaker. Tools and machinery that generate high levels of electromagnetic fields, such as generators and welders, may cause interference with your pacemaker. If you work near such equipment, talk to your cardiologist about having the magnetic field in your workplace measured to determine if you are safe to be near them. Cell phones do not pose a problem, but it is reasonable to hold your cell phone against the ear on the opposite side of your pacemaker. When you are completed with your call, place the pacemaker back on a belt holster or in your purse rather than directly in the breast pocket over your pacemaker. Keep small magnets, such as stereo speakers and magnetic bracelets at least 6 inches away from your pacemaker. If you are a hunter, you may want to talk to your doctor about implanting the pacemaker on the opposite side of your chest so that the recoil of the rifle does not damage your pacemaker's sensitive circuit boards. During some dental and surgical procedures, electric tools are used to stop bleeding. These may also interfere with your pacemaker, and your dentist or surgeon must know that you have a pacemaker prior to any operation. Proceeding through metal detectors is safe for you and your pacemaker. However, the amount of metal in your device may trip the metal detector alarm, and you should be sure to have your pacemaker identification card with you.

I need a defibrillator

Q:?? What is ventricular fibrillation?

Defibrillators are electronic devices that treat ventricular fibrillation. Ventricular fibrillation is a very common rhythm disturbance that costs the lives of about half of patients who die from heart disease, or as many as 350,000 individuals each year. Basically, the heart is composed of millions of individual heart muscle cells. It is the job of the electrical system to stimulate each individual cell simultaneously so that the whole heart contracts together. In fibrillation, each heart cell contracts independently. It's like each instrument in a symphony orchestra playing its own song. The resulting stimulation of the heart muscle produces a quivering action that is incapable of pumping blood. We are all tragically familiar with the occurrence of these arrhythmias. Patients with ventricular fibrillation are often feeling fine and suddenly collapse. Untreated, ventricular fibrillation is usually fatal.

Q:?? What is a defibrillator?

A defibrillator is a machine that delivers an electrical shock through the chest to terminate ventricular fibrillation. Defibrillators have been available in the coronary care units of hospitals for several decades, and are more recently available in ambulances and as free-standing units placed in public buildings. The machine delivers a shock to the patient through paddles applied to the outside of the chest. When used promptly, defibrillation is very successful. However, defibrillators pose two significant problems. First, about 70% of episodes of ventricular fibrillation occur when people are alone. Therefore, no one is aware that a victim requires help. Secondly, although defibrillators are very effective when used promptly, a 10% reduction in success occurs for every one minute of delay in their use. Thus, success rates are high if fibrillation of the heart occurs where a defibrillator is immediately available. However, success rates plummet drastically if a significant delay is required to transport a defibrillator to a victim. For these reasons, defibrillators have now been developed that are small enough to implant inside the body. The implantable type of defibrillator is called an "implantable cardioverter-defibrillator", or ICD.

An ICD has four functions: (1) sensing of the electrical signals in your heart; (2)detection of cardiac rhythm changes; (3)delivery of a shock to terminate ventricular fibrillation; and (4)pacing for slow heart rates. Implanted defibrillators function just as external defibrillators do except that they are entirely automated. When fibrillation is sensed, the device charges a capacitor inside the device and delivers a palpable shock to the heart. Most patients describe the shock as if a fist hit them in the middle of their chest. It is an uncomfortable but instantaneous sensation.

Q:?? What are the benefits of a defibrillator

Studies have now concluded that appropriate patients receiving a defibrillator live longer than similar patients who do not have a defibrillator. Candidates for defibrillators include patients who have already survived a cardiac arrest and those who are at risk of one in the future. Almost everyone who has already survived a cardiac arrest should receive a defibrillator unless the cause of the arrest can be easily recognized and reversed. We also recommend a defibrillator for those who are at high risk of a cardiac arrest in the future. Patients who are at highest risk are those with a significantly weakened heart muscle. We often use an ejection fraction as a marker to identify an appropriate ICD candidate. The ejection fraction is the percentage of blood that the heart ejects with each heartbeat. The normal value is between 55 and 65%. This means that when the heart is full of blood, it will eject about 60% of it with the next heartbeat. When the ejection fraction drifts below 30 to 35%, the risk of a cardiac arrest increases significantly and a defibrillator should be considered. Sometimes, abnormal heart rhythm can lead to a cardiac arrest even in a structurally normal heart. For example, patients with long QT syndrome and Brugada syndrome, discussed in later chapters, may benefit from a defibrillator. Studies indicate that more than one third of appropriately selected patients will receive a shock within two years after ICD implantation.

Q:?? How is a defibrillator implanted?

The defibrillator has two parts, including the generator and the leads. The generator is a small can measuring about 2 x 2 inches, and about half an inch thick. It is composed of a battery and electronic circuit boards. The generator is placed beneath the skin just below the collarbone, and is connected to wires, called leads. The leads are threaded through blood veins into the heart. The generator recognizes the presence of ventricular fibrillation and delivers electricity from the battery to the patient. The leads carry information about the heart's rhythm to the generator, and deliver the shock to the lower chamber if ventricular fibrillation occurs. Following placement of the generator and leads, ventricular fibrillation is often created in the heart muscle to test the system. An external defibrillator is immediately available if the implanted device does not work properly.

Q:?? What complications can occur with a defibrillator?

The most common problem in patients with defibrillators is inappropriate shocks. The ICD measures heart rate to determine when a shock should be delivered. Unfortunately, patients who are extremely anxious or vigorously active can have a normal heartbeat that may exceed this trigger point, resulting in an inappropriate shock. Non-life-threatening arrhythmias of the heart such as atrial fibrillation can also cause the heart to race and trigger inappropriate shocks. In addition, defibrillators may develop manufacturing defects, some of which may result in inappropriate shocks. Advisories and recalls have resulted from defective batteries, defective circuit boards, and problems with the function of the wires. Some of these defects have resulted in inappropriate shocks. Reprogramming the function of the defibrillator can resolve some of these defects. At times, surgery is required to replace the generator or defective lead. Regardless of the cause for inappropriate shocks, be reassured that inappropriate shocks, although very alarming, rarely cause injury to you or your heart. Work with a physician specializing in defibrillator function (called an electrophysiologist) to identify the best treatment to avoid shocks, while being assured that your ICD will function for you when required.

Other complications that can occur during or after defibrillator implantation include infection, a puncture to the lung, or dislodgment of the leads in the first few hours or days after implantation. In general, infection needs to be treated by removal of the entire system and appropriate antibiotic therapy. A puncture of the lung is treated with a small tube placed between the ribs for a few days to evacuate air so that healing can occur. Dislodgment means that the leads become loose from their original location. To correct the problem, the incision usually needs to be reopened so the leads can be placed in a more satisfactory position. Rare complications of ICD implantation include perforation of the heart muscle, bleeding, and shock. Overall, the complications at implantation should not exceed 1 to 2%. Despite all of these possible complications, the probability of being alive with a defibrillator far exceeds survival without one.

Q:?? Will my defibrillator be reliable?

No device as complex as an implantable defibrillator can be totally free of design, manufacturing, and performance flaws. Malfunctions inevitably occur. The leads, or wires connecting the ICD with your heart, have especially been subject to problems. They must withstand the constant beating of the heart, be able to suddenly conduct large voltages of electricity, and perform for years in a body that tries to destroy foreign invaders. Although it is reasonable to expect rare, random failures, ICDs have been subject to more frequent failures that have led to unnecessary shocks, failure to defibrillate, and occasionally death. When the failure rate of an ICD exceeds the industry standard, an advisory is often placed requiring specific action. If the failure rate exceeds the risk of device replacement, a recall may be ordered. Should this happen to your device, frank discussion with an expert in device management will be necessary to explore your options. It is never possible to approach every patient's situation in the same way. You will need to carefully consider the risk of device malfunction and compare it carefully to the risks of device replacement. In many circumstances, a second opinion may be a good option for you.

Q:?? What is a biventricular defibrillator?

Some patients have an electrical problem with their heart called bundle branch block. In this disorder, the two ventricles don't contract at the same time. This distorts the normal geometry of the heart and decreases the amount of blood that it can pump. If you have a bundle branch block and need a defibrillator, you may be a candidate to have a biventricular defibrillator implanted. The biventricular defibrillator has an additional lead that is threaded from the right side of the heart through a blood vein call the coronary sinus that goes over to the left side of the heart. The wires are then hooked up together to the pacemaker so that the right and the left ventricles can beat simultaneously. About 80% of people with a biventricular system feel better with improved exercise capacity. If you have symptoms and are considering implantation of a defibrillator, you may want to talk to your doctor about a biventricular device. Not all patients are candidates and appropriate patient selection is crucial in order to guarantee good results.

Q:?? How will having a defibrillator change my life?

In most instances, having a defibrillator implanted in your chest will have no impact on your lifestyle. Although the size of defibrillators has decreased remarkably over the last few years, they are still somewhat large and in small people may produce a bulge and modest discomfort during vigorous exercise. Few restrictions in your activity should be necessary after your defibrillator except those that are imposed on you by your heart disease. Shortly after implantation, you may be asked to restrict motion of your arm. Unrestricted activities are usually allowed within one to two weeks. Hunters may choose to have their device implanted on the opposite side of the chest, since the recoil of a rifle can damage the device. Otherwise, the device should pose no significant restrictions.

An implanted defibrillator requires regular evaluation. All patients should receive periodic follow-up by an ICD specialist every three to six months. This visit assesses the integrity of the lead, the circuit boards, and the remaining life of the battery. The ICD also stores a record of arrhythmias that have been detected and therapies delivered. Some ICDs also store that may be useful to your doctor. Newer devices can be checked at home through the phone or on the internet. Be sure to discuss the various options available in the follow-up of your particular defibrillator with your physician.

At some point during the follow-up of your device, the battery will begin to deplete and require replacement. During replacement, only the generator is removed and replaced. The leads are generally left in place and will hook up to the new device.

Your defibrillator is constantly searching for ventricular fibrillation. On rare occasions, it may see environmental noise produced by machinery or other electrical sources in your environment and misinterpret it as cardiac activity. In the section of this book dealing with cardiac pacemakers, these interactions were discussed in more detail. The same precautions apply to defibrillators as they due to pacemakers, and you should read this section carefully to understand how to protect your defibrillator from being influenced by environmental noise.

Q:?? What do I do if I receive a shock from my defibrillator?

Most studies report that about one in three patients with a defibrillator will have a shock within the first two years of implantation. Patients who experience a shock and feel well thereafter can be reassured and do not require emergency evaluation. Call your cardiologist responsible for your ICD follow-up to let them know. Patients who experience a shock but do not feel well after the event or who receive more than one shock on the same day require emergency evaluation. A metabolic problem such as low potassium may be aggravating your arrhythmia, or the defibrillator may be malfunctioning. These problems can best be detected and treated in the emergency department of your hospital.

Q:?? Can tones be heard from my defibrillator?

Don't think you're crazy if you think you hear tones coming from your defibrillator. An ICD regularly and automatically checks its own function. If it detects low battery voltage or believes a defect may exist in one of the circuits, your device will emit beeping sounds. These problems are assessed by interrogating your device with a computer and should be done promptly. When your device is first implanted, ask your doctor to let you hear these beeps so that you will recognize them in the future.

Q:?? Can I safely drive with my defibrillator?

Patients with ICDs are understandably concerned about driving restrictions since personal and public safety may be at stake. Because of discomfort at the incision site after a defibrillator implant, it is reasonable for all patients to avoid driving for 5 to 7 days. Thereafter, no highly regarded scientific studies exist to guide our recommendations. However, guidelines from the best experts in the field suggest that driving should not be restricted after the first week or so unless a shock has occurred in the past six months. These recommendations do not apply to the licensing of commercial drivers. According to guidelines published by the U.S. Department of Transportation, ICD implantation disallows certification regardless of the indication for the defibrillator.

Medication for Heart Disease

Placing a name to a medication is a very complex process and defies any easy explanation. Three different names are given to medications. The first is a group name that describes the basic action of the medication. Many different medications may all belong to the same group, and any one medication may belong to several groups depending on the drug's different actions. An example of a drug group is "anticoagulants", or blood thinners. Members of this group include warfarin (Coumadin), aspirin, and clopidogrel (Plavix). The second name given to the medication is its generic name. This name is often complex, long, and barely understandable! Examples include carvedilol and candesartan. The third name is the trade name, given to the drug by the pharmaceutical company that develops and markets it. Each medication has only one generic name, but may have more than one trade name. Thus, discussing drugs in a book dedicated to simplicity becomes extremely challenging! We have chosen to use the generic name in this book followed by common trade names included in parentheses.

Cardiovascular drugs by drug groups:

Anticoagulants (blood thinners)

Anticoagulants are medicines that inhibit our ability to clot blood. Blood thinners do not dissolve clot. The body has its own mechanism to dissolve clot. However, in some conditions our body clots blood faster than we can dissolve it. Therefore, clot accumulates. If blood clotting is a risk for you, blood thinners, or anticoagulants may be necessary to reduce that risk.

Warfarin is a potent blood thinner. The major indications for warfarin are to prevent blood clots in atrial fibrillation, prosthetic heart valve replacements, and blood clots deep in the veins of the legs and pelvis. Warfarin works by depleting the body of vitamin K, a principal building block for blood clotting substances. The effect of warfarin needs to be monitored very carefully, since it is ineffective if the blood is not thin enough yet can cause bleeding if the dose is excessive. In order to monitor warfarin therapy, a blood test is performed called and international normalized ratio, or INR. The normal value for an INR test is less than 1.5. For patients with blood clots or atrial fibrillation, the dose of warfarin should be adjusted to achieve an INR between two and three. For patients with mechanical valve replacements, warfarin should be administered to achieve an INR between 2.5 and 3.5. Initially, INR blood tests are done frequently until the INR is in the right range. The frequency of the INR is then decreased to weekly, then every two weeks, and finally to every month as the INR stabilizes in the desirable range. It is very important to continue INR testing, since patients who have been on warfarin for months or years may suddenly exhibit a need to change their warfarin doses.

Both the food we eat and other medications that we take may influence the amount of warfarin that is prescribed to properly thin the blood. The list of medications that interacts with warfarin is a long one. In short, assume that any new medication you are prescribed may either increase or decrease the amount of warfarin that you take. Whenever you begin a new medication, always ask the prescribing doctor whether it will interact with warfarin, and whether your warfarin dose should change. If so, an INR test may be necessary to be sure your blood tests remain in the right range. Much of our food that we eat contains vitamin K and its intake can also change your warfarin dose. Vitamin K is present in fresh, leafy green vegetables and many fruits. These foods should be kept to a modest amount in your diet. More importantly, the amount you eat needs to be fairly constant over time. It is then possible to adjust the dose of warfarin to accommodate your dietary preferences. However, it will be very difficult to stabilize your warfarin dose if your vitamin K intake varies a lot from day to day.

Q:?? What do I do if I have bleeding while on warfarin?

Many patients who take warfarin have occasional bleeding from their gums when brushing their teeth, or occasional black and blue spots on their skin. However, blood in the urine or stool and coughing up blood are not normal, and the cause for this bleeding should be vigorously evaluated. If you suddenly notice excessive or unusual bleeding, obtain an INR blood test immediately. If the value is high, it will be necessary to discontinue warfarin for a few days to correct the INR. If bleeding is excessive or the INR is very high, your physician may elect to reverse the effects of warfarin by giving you vitamin K orally. It is a good idea to have a few pills of vitamin K available to you at home in case urgent reversal is necessary. Vitamin K comes in a dose of 5 mg. A dose of 2.5 mg often reverses a high INR in 24 hours. Excessively high doses of vitamin K should be used cautiously since it may take several days for the INR to again come up into the therapeutic range.

Q:?? What do I do if I need to stop warfarin for surgery?

It may be necessary to stop warfarin if you need major surgery. However, this doesn't always hold, and is not commonly needed for dental procedures, cataract extractions, skin procedures, and many endoscopies. Therefore, ask your dentist or surgeon first before stopping anticoagulants. If they must be stopped, talk to your cardiologist about the risks of developing a clot. In most cases, some other strategy should be used to thin the blood if you are at high risk. Options include admission to the hospital for intravenous blood thinners such as heparin, or treatment at home with self-administered injections of blood thinners such as enoxaparin (Lovenox).

Anti-Platelet Drugs

Platelets are small, sticky cells that circulate within our bloodstreams, and are very important in the development of clot. Reducing platelet stickiness will still allow a clot to form, but more slowly and less aggressively. Aspirin is perhaps the most well known antiplatelet drug, and is often augmented by the use of clopidogrel (Plavix). Clopidogrel operates in the fashion similar to aspirin, but has a more potent affect inhibiting the formation of clots in the body. The combination of aspirin and clopidogrel is often used to prevent clots following the placement of stents in the coronary arteries. Aspirin and clopidogrel have minimal systemic effects other than bleeding, although allergies can develop to either drug. Blood thinning from both of these drugs begins virtually immediately after ingesting them, and lasts about two weeks after they are stopped. In men, a dose of 81 mg of aspirin daily is usually effective in inhibiting the clotting process, and doses higher than 325 mg are usually not helpful. Women may be more resistant to the effects of aspirin, and 162 to 325 mg of aspirin is often advocated. The maintenance dose for clopidigrel is usually 75mg daily. Other antiplatelet drugs include cilostazol (Pletal) and ticlodipine (Ticlid), usually used to treat symptoms due to impaired circulation of blood in the legs.

Angiotensin-converting enzyme inhibitors (ACE inhibitors)

The kidneys have two functions. One is to filter the blood of unwanted chemicals made during normal metabolism and excrete them into the urine. The second function is to regulate blood pressure. The kidney can sense the pressure of blood flowing through it and excrete an enzyme into the blood stream called angiotensin to correct the blood pressure. Angiotensin, amongst other functions, retains salt and constricts blood vessels, increasing the blood pressure. Therefore, inhibiting angiotensin activity decreases blood pressure. Angiotensin is made from ACE (angiotensin converting enzyme), and inhibiting ACE reduces angiotensin release from the kidneys.

ACE inhibitors are used to treat both high blood pressure and heart failure. High blood pressure responds because the blood vessels in the body dilate and the volume of blood in the system decreases. In heart failure, low blood flow through the kidneys causes angiotensin to be released and promotes salt and water retention. It also constricts blood vessels. This is very deleterious to heart function since more blood needs to be pumped through smaller blood vessels, increasing the work of the heart. Angiotensin converting enzyme inhibitors (or ACEIs), help heart failure patients by reducing angiotensin production and minimizing all of its deleterious effects.

ACE inhibitors are effective and well tolerated medicines. Blood pressure can sometimes decrease too much, resulting in lightheadedness and weakness. Kidney function and potassium levels can occasionally be adversely affected. It is reasonable to obtain kidney function and potassium blood levels shortly after beginning ACE inhibitors. Allergic reactions can also occur, causing rash or dry cough. The cough can be very annoying, and refractory to any management except discontinuation of ACE inhibitors. ACE inhibitors should not be used in pregnancy or in women of child-bearing years since the drugs may cause birth defects in children.

Currently available ACE inhibitors include:

Generic name	Trade name
Enalapril	Vasotec
Captopril	Capoten
Lisinopril	Zestril/Prinivil
Ramipril	Altace
Benazepril	Lotensin
Fosinopril	Monopril
Perindopril	Aceon
Quinapril	Accupril
Trandolapril	Mavik,Tarka
Moexipril	Univasc

Angiotensin receptor blockers

Angiotensin receptor blockers are similar to ACE inhibitors. These drugs block the receptors in the blood vessels where the angiotensin converting enzyme works. The result is very similar. Angiotensin receptor blockers may be used as first line drugs for high blood pressure and heart failure, but are often used when ACE inhibitors can't be used due to side effects. Like ACE inhibitors, these drugs have been shown to reduce the risk of heart failure and save lives. They also have been shown to reduce damage in tissues such as the kidney and brain, especially in hypertensive diabetics. They also may decrease somewhat the occurrence of atrial fibrillation, especially in patients with impaired heart muscle function.

Commonly used angiotensin receptor blockers include:

Generic name	Trade name
Losartan	Cozaar
Candesartan	Atacand
Valsartan	Diovan
Eprosartan	Tevetan
Olmesartan	Benicar
Telmisartan	Micardis
Irbesartan	Avapro

Beta-blockers

Many functions in our bodies occur without us thinking about them. Examples include heart rate, blood pressure control, and the control of our blood vessels. These functions are controlled by the autonomic nervous system. In some sense, we can think of this as the "automatic" nervous system. The autonomic nervous system is composed of two parts. One part is the accelerator, and the other is the brake. The official term for the accelerator is the beta sympathetic arm of the autonomic nervous system. The official term for the brake is the cholinergic arm of the autonomic nervous system. The sympathetic nervous system causes our heart rates to accelerate, our pupils to dilate, and the small hairs in our skin to become upright. A surge of beta sympathetic activity is often referred to as a "flight and fight response." Beta-blockers inhibit the activity of the sympathetic nervous system. As such, beta-blockers lower heart rate and blood pressure at rest and during exercise. Beta-blockers are used to treat high blood pressure and abnormally fast heart rates.

Beta-blockers are generally well tolerated and safe, but occasional side effects may occur such as fatigue and tiredness. Sexual dysfunction is an occasional complaint, particularly in men. Patients with asthma should use caution with beta blockers since their breathing may worsen. On occasion, the heart rate or blood pressure may increase dramatically if beta-blockers are stopped suddenly. It is therefore important to continue this medication and ask your doctor for specific recommendations if the medicine must be stopped. In some situations, it is desirable to slowly taper off of beta-blockers rather than stop them suddenly. If you take insulin or need allergy desensitization shots, be sure that your doctor knows that you are taking beta blockers.

Commonly used beta blockers include:

Generic name	Trade name
Acebutolol	Sectral
Atenolol	Tenormin
Betoxolol	Kerlone
Carvedilol	Coreg
Metoprolol	Lopressor, Toprol
Propranolol	Inderal
Nadolol	Corgard
Timolol	Blocadren

Lipid-lowering Drugs:

Q:?? What are statin drugs?

Statins are powerful medications used to treat high cholesterol. These drugs can often reduce the cholesterol level in half! They have clearly been demonstrated to reduce the risk of heart attack, stroke, and reduce the rate of acceleration of arteriosclerosis. Statins also reduce the inflammation seen in the lining of our blood vessels that predisposes us to hardening of the arteries. Statins also reduce serious cardiac arrhythmias that can result in sudden, unexpected death.

Several statin drugs are now available, and can result in two common side effects. Liver function is measured by elevations in liver enzymes measured in the blood stream, and may rarely become effected on statin drugs. Some clinicians prefer to continue statin drugs despite slight liver abnormalities and have observed that the elevations frequently become normal on their own in time. Liver enzymes should be obtained once or twice yearly in all patients who use statin medication.

Muscle inflammation is the more troublesome side effect with statins, and occurs in from 2 to 3% of patients. The usual complaint is muscle soreness or weakness beginning usually within the first four months of treatment. Fortunately, diagnosing muscular inflammation from statin drugs is easy since the symptoms improve quickly soon after the drugs are stopped. A variety of approaches can be used when statin drugs are felt to be essential in patients who have exhibited muscular inflammation. Several weeks off the drugs may be required for the inflammation to totally subside. Thereafter, a different statin can be started in very low dose, and gradually increased to a more therapeutic level.

Commonly used statin drugs include:

Generic name	Trade name
Simvastatin	Zocor
Rosuvastatin	Crestor
Atorvostatin	Lipitor
Fluvastatin	Lescol
Lovastatin	Mevacor, Altoprev
Pravastatin	Pravachol

Non-statin alternatives for cholesterol reduction

Statin medications are considered the drugs of choice to lower cholesterol. However, some patients do not tolerate statins well, usually due to sore muscles. Most non-statin alternatives to lower cholesterol work by inhibiting the absorption of cholesterol from the intestines. Examples include cholesterol absorption inhibitors, fibrates, and bile acid binding drugs. An example of a drug that inhibits cholesterol absorption is ezetimibe (Zetia). Bile acid binding drugs include cholestyramine (Questran), colestipol (Colestid), and colesevelam (WelChol). These drugs work in the intestines to increase your excretion of cholesterol. Fibrates are used to lower triglycerides and may raise the HDL. With the exception of gemfibrozil, they can be used along with statin drugs for a better effect. Examples include gemfibrozil (Lopid), fenofibrate (Antara, Lofibra, Tricor, and Triglide),and clofibrate (Atromid). Niacin can also be helpful in reducing LDL cholesterol and increasing HDL cholesterol.

Non-statin drugs are usually well tolerated, and rarely cause muscular soreness like the statin drugs. The major side effects are stomach upset, diarrhea, nausea, and abdominal bloating. Niacin can cause intolerable skin flushing in some patients. The long-acting forms or slow release forms of niacin may be better tolerated, and the flushing effect of niacin may be blocked by taking aspirin one hour before niacin.

Vasodilators

Vasodilators are medications that dilate arterial blood vessels. They reduce blood pressure and reduce the amount of work the heart must do to pump blood. The most common indications for vasodilators are hypertension and heart failure. Vasodilators tend not to be used as first-line drugs for the management of hypertension. In heart failure, vasodilators are third line drugs to be used only when angiotensin converting enzyme inhibitors or angiotensin receptor blockers are not effective. Hydralazine as an example of a vasodilator used to treat hypertension.

Vasodilators are generally well tolerated medications with few serious side effects. Hydralazine may result in an unusual inflammatory disease similar to lupus. This reaction is uncommon, and accompanied by rash, fever, and arthritis. The lupus-like condition caused by hydralazine usually goes away quickly when the drug is discontinued.

Digoxin

Digoxin is one of the earliest cardiac medications used to treat heart patients. It has two major effects, including slowing of the heart rate and strengthening of the heart contraction. It is usually used to control the rate when rapid arrhythmias cause the heart to race. However, digoxin controls heart rate at rest better than it does during exercise. Digoxin has also been used for decades to treat heart failure by improving the hearts contractility, but its effectiveness is modest at best. Some studies have suggested that digoxin may worsen the outlook of patients with heart failure, and it has therefore lost much its prior appeal.

Side effects to digoxin are rare unless blood levels become excessive. If levels are too high, digoxin may cause slowing of the heart rate, nausea, and vomiting. Some evidence suggests that sudden withdrawal of digoxin in heart failure patients may precipitate acute worsening of heart failure. If you have kidney disease, your dose of digoxin may need to be reduced since digoxin is removed from the body through the kidneys. Blood levels of digoxin can be monitored to determine the correct dose for you.

Digoxin may interact with several other medications. Amiodarone and calcium channel blockers such as diltiazem and verapamil may increase the blood level of digoxin. Antacids and Kaopectate may decrease the absorption of digoxin, and should be used only several hours before or after digoxin is taken. Cholestyramine and colestipol may decrease the absorption of digoxin. These drugs should not be used together.

Nitrates

Nitrates have many actions that may be useful in alleviating chest pain in people with coronary artery disease. Nitrates dilate the veins of the body and may reduce the workload of the heart. They dilate the arteries to the heart, improving blood supply. Nitrates come in several forms, including a paste on the skin, patches, pills and capsules, and a spray or small pills to be used under the tongue. Nitroglycerin in either a spray form or a small pill under the tongue should be given to all patients who have chest pain from their heart or have had a prior heart attack. The spray has a longer shelf life and slightly faster onset of action. Nitroglycerin pills have a relatively short shelf life, and should be replaced at least annually. Long-acting forms of nitroglycerin pills or capsules can provide relief of chest pain and improve exercise capacity. Examples include isosorbide dinitrate taken two or 3 times daily, and isosorbide mononitrate, taken once daily. Nitroglycerin also comes in a patch placed randomly on the skin every day. Some patients may become tolerant to nitroglycerin when placed on the skin, and notice less effect when used day after day. If you use a nitroglycerin patch, talk to your doctor about interrupting therapy. Patients who regularly experience chest discomfort on exertion during daytime hours can place the patch on each morning, and remove it at bedtime. Some patients who present with chest pain awakening them from sleep at night could benefit from nitroglycerin patches placed at bedtime and taken off in the morning.

Diuretics

Diuretics, or water pills, increase the excretion of water from the body. Two groups of diuretics are commonly used. One group is called thiazide diuretics. Examples include hydrochlorothiazide, and chlorthalidone. The second type of diuretic is called a loop diuretic. Examples include furosemide (Lasix), torsemide (Demadex), and bumetanide (Bumex). Diuretics are used to treat hypertension and heart failure. In hypertension, thiazide diuretics are usually used to reduce overall blood volume. By reducing volume, the pressure in the system drops. Loop diuretics are more powerful, and are usually used only in patients who fail to respond to thiazide diuretics. Most patients with heart failure also require loop diuretics.

If you have heart failure, talk to your doctor about modifying your diuretic dose on a daily basis according to changes in your body fluids.

Watch carefully for changes in body weight, swelling, and shortness of breath. A good way to detect swelling is to press on the shin bone for 3 to 5 seconds. When you release your finger, you should not be able to feel any indentation in the spot where you were pressing. A persistent indentation means swelling is present. Another sensitive indicator of retained fluid is a sudden increase in your weight. All patients with heart failure should weigh themselves daily, in the morning, with no clothes on. For most of us, our body weight each morning does not vary by more than about two pounds. Therefore, more than a two pound gain usually reflects fluid accumulation. Depending upon your sensitivity to diuretics, you can increase your diuretic dose to get rid of water before it becomes a problem for you. For example, many patients may require 40 mg of furosemide each day to manage their fluid. If you observe a three pound weight gain and slight edema you would respond by increasing the daily dose to 80 mg for 3 days, thereafter returning to your 40-mg dose. The exact doses you will require need to be worked out with your physician. This is a very successful method for you to help manage your own chronic disease.

Diuretics are double-edged swords, and can cause dehydration if used injudiciously, or if another source of fluid loss occurs such as diarrhea or fever. Dehydration is suspected if you feel lightheaded when you stand quickly or excessive thirst. Diuretics can also cause abnormalities in kidney function and reduce your blood potassium level. Potassium levels should be measured a few days after beginning a diuretic to determine whether potassium supplementation is needed. Although fresh fruits such as bananas contain some potassium, they often fall short of supplying enough potassium to meet the needs of patients on loop diuretics.

Anti-arrhythmic (cardiac rhythm controlling) drugs

Anti-rhythmic drugs are medications that help to restore a normal rhythm to the heart and prevent their recurrence. Examples include sotalol, flecainide, dofetilide, amiodarone, propafenone, quinidine, and procainamide. For the most part, these medications are used to prevent arrhythmias coming from the upper chambers of the heart, such as supraventricular tachycardia and atrial fibrillation or atrial flutter. For arrhythmias that are infrequent, these medications can by used as a "pill in the pocket." Using this method, an anti-arrhythmic drug such as propafenone is taken as soon as you feel the onset of an abnormal rhythm, and the drug does not need to be taken for the weeks or months between arrhythmias.

The most serious side effect of anti-rhythmic drugs is called pro-arrhythmic effect. This means that a drug designed to suppress abnormal rhythms can actually create new and worse arrhythmia. Particularly those arrhythmias arising in the lower chamber of the heart can worsen with anti-rhythmic drug treatment, and can be very dangerous. An increase in sudden death in patients taking anti-rhythmic drugs has been documented.

Amiodarone deserves special consideration relative to its side effects. When used in high doses over a long time, this drug can cause scarring of the lungs, abnormal thyroid function and deterioration in liver function. . Amiodarone can also cause a blue-gray discoloration of the skin, tremor, and numbness of the hands or feet due to neuropathy. Its main use is in the short term prevention of atrial fibrillation after heart surgery, and to suppress dangerous rhythm disturbances from the lower chambers of the heart that trigger frequent shocks from an implanted defibrillator. If used beyond a brief time, liver tests, thyroid tests, and evaluation of lung function should be done at least every six months. If you are receiving long-term amiodarone for non-life threatening arrhythmias, talk to your doctor about other alternatives with less toxic medication or consider ablation procedures to cure your arrhythmia.

Dofetilide is a rhythm controlling medication that helps control atrial fibrillation. Dofetilide is dosed according to an interval that is measured on the electrocardiogram. Because of this complexity of prescribing the drug and the possibility that the drug can worsen your arrhythmia, it is mandatory to start dofetilide in the hospital. Dofetilide has few side effects and is generally well tolerated. Nausea, skin rash, and headache are infrequently reported.

Propafenone is another rhythm controlling agent that is helpful to prevent atrial fibrillation, atrial flutter, and supraventricular tachycardia. The drug is generally well tolerated, but may cause dizziness, blurred vision, constipation, or skin rash. Use the drug cautiously if you have heart failure, since it may weaken the contraction of the heart muscle.

Both calcium channel blockers and beta blockers are also used to control heart rhythm disturbances and should be considered as anti-arrhythmic agents as well.

Calcium channel blockers

Calcium channel blockers include a large group of drugs that blocker calcium channel activity, important in heart muscle contraction and blood vessel constriction. Calcium channel blockers dilate arterial blood vessels. As such, they are commonly used to treat high blood pressure. Some calcium channel blockers, such as diltiazem and verapamil, also slow heart rate, and they may be helpful in the management of fast cardiac rhythm disturbances. Some calcium channel blockers such as amlodipine do not affect heart rate, and may be more helpful in the management of hypertension if heart rates are somewhat low. Calcium channel blockers can also be used to treat patients with chest pain due to angina by dilating the blood vessels to the heart.

Calcium channel blockers are generally well tolerated with a low incidence of serious side effects. Amlodipine may cause occasional swelling in the legs. Verapamil may slow the heart rate and cause constipation. Diltiazem is generally better tolerated, with only modest constipation. If you have had a coronary stent placed in the past, remember that calcium blockers may decrease the favorable effects of clopidogrel (Plavix) in keeping stents from clotting closed. Talk to your doctor to see if an alternative is available.

Examples of calcium channel blockers include diltiazem, amlodipine, nifedipine, nicardipine and verapamil. Side effects include worsening of heart failure, slowing of heart rate, and constipation. Nicardipine, amlodipine, and nifedipine do not slow the heart rate and are used to treat hypertension and chest discomfort in patients with angina. Side effects are similar to other calcium channel blockers, but swelling of the feet may be a particular problem with nifedipine and amlodipine.

Calcium channel blockers include:

Generic Name	Trade Name
Amlodipine	Norvasc, Lotrel
Bepridil	Vascor
Diltiazem	Cardizem, Tiazac, Cartia, Dilacor
Felodipine	Plendil
Nisoldipine	Sular
Verapamil	Calan, Covera, Isoptin, Verelan

Q:?? What is combination drug therapy?

A few drugs are marketed in combination with another drug. For instance, Tenoretic is a combination of a beta blocker called atenolol (Tenormin) and chlorthalidone, a diuretic. Using combination drugs reduces the number of pills you need to take each day, and may be slightly less expensive. However, they do sometimes interfere with the ability to titrate both drugs carefully. Speak with your doctor about avoiding combination drugs until your dose of each agent has been proven to be effective and well tolerated. Thereafter, switching the two drugs to a combination agent may be worthwhile.

Q:?? When should I take my medication?

Compliance is a term the medical profession uses to describe the accuracy with which patients take their medication. Few of us to take our medication exactly right all the time. Some hints to help you improve your compliance include:

- Establish a routine and always take your medication at the same time each day.
- Try to take your medication at a routine time such as breakfast or bedtime.
- Use a pill planner. This is a small box to organize your daily medication.
- If you must take a medicine at an unusual time of day, consider a wrist watch that has an alarm to remind you.

High blood pressure medication may be more effective when taken at bedtime when our bodies are naturally repairing themselves.

Grapefruit juice may decrease the absorption some of your medications. It is not clear how much grapefruit juice is required to interfere with medicines or for how long the effect lasts. In addition, different medications may be more or less affected by the ingestion of grapefruit juice. Until all of these issues are better understood, it is probably reasonable to avoid drinking grapefruit juice if you use cardiovascular medication.

I'm having an angioplasty

Q:?? What is angioplasty

Coronary angioplasty is a technique to repair a blockage in an artery. It is most commonly applied to a coronary artery but can be used in other arteries such as the carotid or kidney artery. In most instances, angioplasty is performed with a high pressure balloon. The balloon is gradually advanced through the area of blockage. With the balloon crossing the blockage, it is inflated using a high pressure inflator. In most instances, the relatively soft and compressible material that creates blockage is compressed, leaving behind minimal residual blockage.

Q:?? How is angioplasty performed?

Angioplasty helps improve blood supply to the heart muscle. It has two indications. Many patients have serious symptoms such as chest pain or shortness of breath that limit their lifestyle. When medications don't improve symptoms, angioplasty may provide significant relief. Secondly, angioplasty may be a life saving maneuver in carefully selected patients. As discussed in the beginning of this book, angioplasty is definitely indicated in most patients with an acute heart attack. It is also helpful for patients who have highly threatening blockages in one of the major blood vessels such as the left anterior descending artery on the front wall of the heart. However, many patients will respond equally well or even better when treated with medication alone. If you are feeling well with little or no chest pain or shortness of breath and have a blockage in a blood vessel other than the left anterior descending artery, talk to your doctor about obtaining another opinion before proceeding with an elective angioplasty.

Q:?? What risks occur during angioplasty?

As with all procedures done inside the body, angioplasty has risk. About one in one hundred patients will have a serious complication or not survive the procedure. This risk will vary depending upon the strength of your heart, the severity of the blockages, and your overall health. Diseases such as diabetes and kidney failure markedly increase the risk of angioplasty. The most commonly encountered complications include heart attack, stroke, bleeding at the site of entry into the blood vessels, allergic reactions to the contrast material, perforation of the blood vessel, and rhythm disturbances of the heart. In good hands, all of these complications together should not exceed 1%.

Q:?? What is a stent?

Under some circumstances, a stent is placed into the coronary artery following angioplasty. A stent is a metallic mesh device measuring less than one inch in length that is placed across the vessel narrowing after angioplasty. When the balloon deploying the stent is inflated, the stent is pushed into the inner lining of the blood vessel and stays open.

Q:?? What is the controversy involving the two kinds of stents?

Two kinds of stents are used during angioplasty. Bare metal stents contain no coating, while drug coated stents have a thin layer of medicine on the metal to reduce scar and blood clot formation within the stent. Numerous studies have focused on which of these stents is better. A consistent finding in all of the studies is that drug-eluting stents significantly reduce the need for future procedures to fix stent-related problems. However, no significant differences in survival or the incidence of heart attack has been consistently noted between the two stents. Blood thinners must be prescribed after all stent placements, but blood thinning is most important with the drug-coated types. Before receiving a stent, you should talk with your doctor about the need for blood thinners following stent placement. You need to confirm with your doctor your willingness to comply with blood thinning therapy. If you are likely to require some form of surgery for which blood thinners must be interrupted during the 12 months following a stent, consider having an angioplasty without stent placement or at least a non-coated stent, since interruption of blood thinning following the placement of a drug-eluting stent is particularly hazardous.

Q:?? What medication must I take after angioplasty?

Continuing aspirin and clopidogrel after a stent is placed in your heart is absolutely necessary. Particularly with drug-coated stents, discontinuation of clopidogrel in the first 3 months following stent placement may cause a heart attack. Oftentimes, advice to stop medication is given by physicians or dentists who are unaware of the dangers of stopping these medicines. We absolutely prohibit discontinuing aspirin or clopidogrel following stent placement for the first 3 months unless a life-threatening emergency requiring surgery occurs. We strongly encourage continuing these medicines through the first year after stent placement. Some experts believe clopidogril should be continued for up to 3 years following angioplasty and stent placement in order to do the best we can to prevent stent clotting.

I need coronary artery bypass surgery.

Q:?? Why should I have coronary bypass surgery?

Understanding the rationale to proceed with coronary artery bypass surgery is always a pressing issue for every patient. Coronary artery bypass surgery is usually recommended for two reasons: surgery improves cardiac symptoms in most patients and it prolongs life in some patients. Improvement in symptoms is reasonably straightforward. Most patients who are restricted by chest pain or shortness of breath feel better with fewer symptoms and a higher exercise capacity after surgery.

Understanding who will live longer after coronary artery bypass surgery is a more complicated issue. When a badly blocked blood vessel occludes, the area of heart muscle supplied by that blood vessel will become damaged. Therefore, it stands to reason that if the blocked blood vessel is large and supplies an important part of heart tissue, a successful bypass will prevent a large heart attack. In contrast, a smaller blood vessel supplying a small amount of heart tissue will pose a less serious risk and may not benefit from bypass. Life expectancy improved after bypass surgery only in a few situations, including left main coronary artery obstruction, obstruction of the left anterior descending coronary artery, and in obstruction of all three major arteries to the heart. However, understand that every persons anatomy of the blood vessels to their heart differs somewhat. The benefit surgery provides patients is a complex issue that needs to be discussed carefully with your doctor. It is one topic that often will benefit by a second opinion.

In summary, bypass surgery may benefit you in the following situations:

- Symptoms of shortness of breath or chest pain exists due to blockages in arteries that limit your activities and do not respond to medication.
- Narrowing exists in your left main coronary artery.
- Narrowing exists in the first portion of your left anterior descending coronary artery.
- Severe narrowing exists in all three arteries supplying your heart, especially if you have impairment in the strength of your heart muscle.

Q:?? How is coronary bypass surgery performed?

When driving in a bad traffic, you may need to drive a few extra blocks to get around the traffic. This is exactly what's done in bypass surgery. The blockage is not removed. Rather, a leg vein is sewn to the aorta, and the other end is sewn onto the coronary artery just beyond the blockage. In most cases, the procedure is done while the heart is still and no longer beating. The blood is oxygenated and circulated by an external bypass machine. In other cases, surgery is done without bypass. The advantages of performing surgery without bypass are not really clear. At one time, losing cognitive skills after bypass surgery was felt to give an advantage to off pump surgery. Recent data does not support this advantage.

Q:?? Why is a LIMA graft important?

The left anterior descending coronary artery is the most important artery of the heart. When it is becomes blocked, maintaining an open bypass for many years becomes important. Rather than using a saphenous vein from the leg for a bypass, surgeons are more commonly using the left internal mammary artery, or LIMA. This artery arises from the left shoulder area and supplies the front chest wall. The end of the vessel is removed from the chest wall and is sewn onto the left anterior descending coronary artery. Studies have shown that left internal mammary artery grafts are more likely to stay open longer than veins taken from the leg. If you have significant narrowing of your left anterior descending coronary artery, you should insist that a LIMA graft be considered in the operative approach to your care.

Q:?? Can bypass surgery cure my heart disease?

Some patients mistakenly believe that their disease is now behind them after surgery. Quite to the contrary, bypass surgery does not fix the disease process that afflicts your arteries. Bypassing around areas of existing blockage simply give you a new lease on life, with more time to dedicate yourself to a better lifestyle. If your lifestyle is not changed, your bypasses will clog up and you will either need another operation in the future or die from a heart attack. The importance of maintaining ideal body weight, eating properly, and being physically active are every bit as important following surgery as they are after your first heart attack.

Q:?? What medication should I go home on following surgery?

All the medication you were prescribed to prevent arteriosclerosis before your operation should be continued afterwards. Minimally, this includes cholesterol-lowering medication, high blood pressure medication, and aspirin. In some patients, blood pressure becomes lower following surgery and high blood pressure medicine may need to be withheld temporarily. However, high blood pressure inevitably returns so keep monitoring your blood pressure carefully. If atrial fibrillation complicated your surgery, as it does an up to one third of patients, rhythm controlling medicines may be briefly necessary after your operation. However, you should discuss with your doctor stopping these drugs two or three months postoperatively.

Chapter 5: Special Situations in Heart Disease

What about women and heart disease?

Cardiovascular disease is a leading health concern for women, and is responsible for half of all deaths in women over age 50 years of age. Unfortunately, much of the scientific information that has been gathered about heart disease has been in men. Several analyses recently suggest that some clinically important differences exist between men and women regarding their heart disease. Some examples include:

- Women with diabetes have a significantly higher cardiovascular risk than men.
- Women with atrial fibrillation are at greater risk of stroke.
- Symptoms reported by women often differ from men.
- Women are less likely than men to receive angioplasty or coronary bypass surgery after a heart attack.
- Short-term mortality for women with chest pain is higher although they may exhibit lower long-term mortality.
- Women appear to have better long-term survival after coronary artery bypass surgery.
- Aspirin after a heart attack is equally effective in women and men, but aspirin used to prevent future heart disease is not as effective in women.
- Prevention using aspirin for stroke reduction is equally effective in women and men.

Sudden cardiac death in athletes

Very few tragedies strike as hard in our hearts as sudden unexpected death in young athletes. In almost all instances, death is caused by a cardiac rhythm disturbance. Hypertrophic cardiomyopathy is the most common cause of these lethal arrhythmias. This inherited disease strikes the heart muscle, causing it to become thickened and overly contractile. In most instances, no symptoms occur until sudden death strikes. Although some individuals will have a family history of unexpected sudden death, victims are usually unaware of their diagnosis. Some individuals will experience palpitations, lightheadedness on exertion or shortness of breath, although symptoms are usually not very spectacular. Some athletes may have been ill with a flu-like syndrome for a few days before their collapse. This disease, called viral cardiomyopathy, causes weakness of the heart muscle and may be complicated by serious and sudden death. Rarer causes of unexpected sudden death in youngsters include congenital abnormalities in the formation of the coronary arteries and genetic abnormalities of cardiac rhythm formation.

The best screening for youngsters about to engage in heavy, competitive athletics remains controversial. When a youngster sees his or her doctor, be prepared to discuss complaints of palpitations of the heart, lightheadedness, episodes of fainting, or discomfort in the chest. Be aware that the physical diagnosis may be entirely normal in youngsters with many of those disorders that result in sudden death. If any question arises about a personal history of heart complaints or a family history of sudden unexpected cardiac death, and electrocardiogram will also be helpful and an echocardiogram may be diagnostic.

What is the Long QT Syndrome

The QT interval is a measurable interval of time that is required for the heart to contract and then relax with each heartbeat. It can be easily seen and measured on the EKG. In some patients, the EKG shows an unusually long QT interval. We find that individuals with this finding are more prone to fainting and sudden, unexplained death. The cause remains unknown, but relates to a defective flow of potassium and sodium in the electrical channels of the heart. The disorder is strongly genetic. The diagnosis is sometimes evident on the EKG, but may be only intermittently present, making the diagnosis very difficult. All patients who faint suddenly and unexpectedly should be evaluated for this diagnosis, particular young females with a family history of sudden death.

Several options exist to treat patients with this diagnosis. In some circumstances, treatment with medicines such as beta blockers is sufficient. In others, a defibrillator should be implanted. In all cases, genetic counseling should be sought, including careful screening of siblings and children of affected patients. Reasonably cost effective genetic testing is now available for patients that may help clarify their risk and the presence of this disease in relatives. However, be careful when investigating genetic testing as the field is progressing extremely rapidly and highly sophisticated opinions should be sought.

What is Marfan Syndrome?

Marfan syndrome is a genetic disease that affects young people. Patients with Marfan syndrome have long arms and legs, thin muscles, and abnormalities of their eyes, lungs, and hearts. Heart defects include mitral valve prolapse and dilatation of the aorta. Many years ago, Marfan syndrome carried a poor outlook, but better survival is now seen with appropriate medical and surgical treatment. All Marfan syndrome patients, regardless of the presence of aortic disease, should be treated with beta blocker drugs. Follow-up needs to be vigorous with frequent evaluations for the cardiovascular complications of the disease.

What is the metabolic syndrome?

The metabolic syndrome is a disturbance of sugar and fat. It is defined as any three of the following five characteristics: abdominal obesity (waist >40 inches in men or >35 inches in women), triglycerides >150mg/dl, HDL (good cholesterol) <40 in men or <50 in women, blood pressure > 130/85mmHg, and fasting glucose > 110mg/dl. These diagnostic criteria are present in up to 47 million adults over the age of 20. The metabolic syndrome is associated a high risk of coronary artery disease.

If you have the metabolic syndrome, you must modify each of its manifestations. Obtaining ideal body weight improves obesity and reduces triglyceride levels. Regular exercise is essential in blood pressure and glucose control. Drugs that increase HDL levels and reduce triglycerides may also be helpful. Patients who properly manage these factors enjoy a markedly reduced chance of diabetes in later life.

Living with an artificial heart valve

A markedly abnormal heart valve may need to be replaced when it starts to produce symptoms or begins to harm the heart. Fortunately, currently used valve replacements function very similarly to normal valves. Two types are currently implanted. A mechanical prosthesis is made entirely of metal or plastic. It is designed to last a normal lifetime, and has a very low incidence of valve dysfunction. Lifetime blood thinning with warfarin is necessary. A second type of prosthesis is called a tissue valve. It is often made from animal tissue such as the pericardium, or the tissue that encases the heart. Some tissue valves may not last a full lifetime and a second valve replacement may be necessary. The main advantage to tissue valves is that blood thinners may not be necessary. You need to carefully discuss these issues with your cardiologist and surgeon and make a careful choice. Remember that warfarin, the blood thinner required for mechanical valves, cannot be used during pregnancy, although alternative intravenous or subcutaneously injected blood thinners may be considered. Young women of child-bearing age should therefore consider this factor.

If you have an artificial heart valve, antibiotics must be taken immediately before any surgical or dental procedures that may result in bacteria entering the bloodstream. Only a single dose is necessary about one hour before the procedure. Be certain to discuss with any doctor or dentist who has asked you to undergo an operation or procedure whether antibiotics are required.

What about sleep apnea?

Sleep apnea is a condition that causes repeated episodes of obstructed breathing during sleep together with daytime sleepiness and altered cardiac and/or lung function. Sleep apnea is very common in our country, currently effecting over 15 million Americans. The prevalence of sleep disturbances rises dramatically in obese subjects. Weight management is essential to adequately manage sleep apnea. From a cardiac viewpoint, patients with sleep apnea have an increased risk of hypertension, cardiac arrhythmias, right and left-sided heart failure, heart attack, and stroke, as well as an overall increased mortality rate. Numerous treatments are available for sleep apnea, but weight loss in obese patients should always be advocated.

Holes in the heart and headache

During the first few weeks after a baby is conceived, the upper half of the heart has only one chamber. Over a course of a few weeks, a wall of tissue grows in the middle of this large chamber, dividing it into two halves. A healthy baby is then born with two separate, completely divided upper chambers to the heart. Some of us are born with a hole in the wall, allowing the communication of blood between the right and left atria. In its worst form, a large defect in the wall may exist, called an atrial septal defect. In less serious cases, only a small communication persists, which is often closed by a small, mobile tissue flap. This small hole has been named a "foramen ovale." Most of the time, the blood pressure in the left atrium is higher than in the right atrium. Any blood flow that courses through the hole therefore usually goes from the left atrium to the right atrium. It is not uncommon that small pieces of blood clot or other debris may travel from various parts of our body back to the right atrium and to the lungs. The lungs are especially equipped to digest particulate debris and rid the body of it. However, on some occasions the pressure in the right atrium may acutely rise. This commonly occurs when we bear down, or have coughing jags or frequent sneezing. If particulate debris happens to be traveling through the right atrium as the pressure suddenly rises, it may float from the right to the left atrium. With the next heartbeat, this debris is then pumped out through the left ventricle to the body. The brain is particularly sensitive to small clots traveling into the blood vessels, and a stroke or severe migraine headache may result.

An echocardiogram, or cardiac ultrasound, will usually identify a patent (or open) foramen ovale, sometimes called a PFO. To increase the yield of an echo, salt water is shaken with a small amount of air so that bubbles can be injected into the blood stream. The echocardiogram detects bubbles traveling from the right atrium into the left atrium through the small PFO. These bubbles are microscopic in size, dissipate quickly, and do not cause any risk to the patient.

Many clinical conditions have been associated with the presence of a PFO. A stroke that has no other apparent cause, called a "cryptogenic stroke," decompression sickness in deep-sea divers, and blood clots traveling throughout the body have all been attributed to PFO. Recently, increasing interest has riveted on an association between PFO and migraine headaches. In some studies, closure of the PFO has been associated with complete resolution of migraine in up to 60% of patients. However, other studies have not confirmed a close relationship between PFO and migraine, with disappointing results after PFO closure.

Options to treat patients with PFO's and neurological events include medical treatment with blood thinners, surgical closure, or closure through a catheter-based device advanced from a groin blood vessel. Complications when closing a PFO by using a catheter have been reduced to approximately 1%, and new techniques are constantly being developed to close PFOs using a non-operative approach. However, no evidence currently exists supporting any treatment for PFO in patients who have no symptoms from its presence.

Indications for antibiotics before surgical procedures

Infective endocarditis is a bacterial infection of one or more of the valves of the heart. Bacteria that gain entry into the blood stream during a surgical or dental procedure may initiate the infection. It is often recommended that antibiotics be used prior to procedures in order to reduce the chance of infection. However, the effectiveness of antibiotic treatment has recently been questioned, and potential harm due to allergic reactions to antibiotics is being increasingly recognized. Therefore, newer recommendations significantly decreased the number of patients and kinds of procedures for which antibiotics are required. We now require that antibiotics be administered only in patients with complex congenital heart disease and in those who have had previous episodes of endocarditis or surgically replaced heart valves. Dental procedures requiring antibiotics should be restricted to those that involve manipulation of the gum tissue or perforation of the skin lining the mouth. Antibiotics are no longer recommended to prevent endocarditis prior to gastrointestinal or genitourinary tract procedures such as colonoscopy or endoscopy. Amoxicillin or ampicillin is still the treatment of choice, taking 2 g orally one hour before the procedure. Consult with your physician for appropriate antibiotic alternatives if you are allergic to penicillin.

What is aortic stenosis?

The aortic valve must fully open as the left ventricle contracts in order that blood can be ejected out to the body. Aortic stenosis is a thickening and stiffening of the aortic valve that prevents it from fully opening. The most common cause of aortic stenosis is a birth defect of the valve called bicuspid aortic stenosis. The aortic valve normally has three tissue flaps attached to it that open and close with every heartbeat. A bicuspid valve has only two flaps, and is prone to become thickened and calcified usually between the ages of 50 and 70. In older individuals, aortic stenosis can also arise from calcium deposition in an otherwise normal valve.

Aortic stenosis produces three symptoms: shortness of breath, chest discomfort, and lightheadedness or fainting. Symptoms usually occur on exertion, and often do not occur until aortic stenosis is quite severe. Once symptoms have developed, surgical replacement of the aortic valve is often required. In the absence of symptoms, aortic stenosis can usually be observed without surgery. The severity of aortic stenosis can be easily assessed by the echocardiogram, which shows both thickening and calcification of the valve, as well as calculates the drop in blood pressure across the valve caused by its stiffness and inability to fully open. The drop in pressure across the valve correlates quite closely with the severity of narrowing. When the drop in blood pressure across the valve exceeds 50 – 60-mm Hg, the valve will have to be followed quite closely for consideration of surgical replacement. For the most part, no treatment is available short of surgery, and no known treatment significantly impacts on the progression of its stiffness. The severity of the valve problem must be watched carefully, and when it becomes severe, and/or symptoms occur, surgical replacement of the valve is indicated.

What is mitral valve prolapse?

Mitral valve prolapse, or MVP, is a common abnormality of the mitral valve that may lead to leakage of blood through the valve. The mitral valve lies between the left atrium and the left ventricle. Blood entering into the left ventricle must pass through the mitral valve. As the ventricle begins its contraction, the mitral valve closes, forcing the blood to exit the left ventricle through the aortic valve and into the aorta. The mitral valve is shaped much like a parachute. Two tissue flaps are attached to the valve by many long cords, called chordae tendinae, that connect to a muscle in the left ventricle. As the muscle contracts, the cords pull the tissue flaps closed. As the muscle relaxes, the cords extend, and the mitral valve opens. In MVP, the tissue flaps are excessively large and floppy. Therefore, when the papillary muscle contracts, the elongated cords cannot pull the redundant tissue flaps closed. Leakage therefore results.

Some patients with mitral valve prolapse complain of palpitations and chest pain. For many years, unexplained chest pain and palpitations were often erroneously attributed to MVP. Clearly, the diagnosis was applied far too often, and many patients who carry a diagnosis of mitral valve prolapse have normal or nearly normal mitral valve structure. If you have been told in the past that you have mitral valve prolapse and are concerned about it, you may wish to revisit this issue with your cardiologist and determine whether the diagnosis can still be established given current diagnostic criteria.

Most people with mitral valve prolapse will live normal lives, and very few develop symptoms or ever need medication or surgery for their condition. A small number may develop leaking through the valve. This condition initially is treated with medications such as ACE inhibitors and diuretics. Antibiotics for MVP are no longer recommended prior to dental or surgical procedures.

I've been told I have a heart murmur. What is that?

A heart murmur is simply a noise that one hears while listening to the heart with a stethoscope. It is caused by unusual turbulence in the flow of blood. A murmur is very analogous to the rapids of a river. If water is flowing smoothly through a riverbed, no noise is generated. However, we hear rapids when large volumes of water roar turbulently downstream. Similarly, blood flow through the heart is also usually quiet and undisturbed. However, at times it may become turbulent producing a murmur. A murmur in and of itself is not diagnostic of a heart problem. Many normal individuals have some turbulence in the flow of their blood through their heart, causing what we call an innocent murmur. Innocent murmurs are often heard during childhood, adolescence, and pregnancy. However, turbulence may also be generated because a valve is sticky, leaky, or a hole is present between the chambers of the heart. In such examples, a heart murmur may indicate a serious underlying structural heart problem.

I have neurocardiogenic syncope. What in the world is that?

A brief lapse in consciousness is called syncope. It is in contrast to coma which involves long lapses in consciousness. Syncope has many causes but one of the most common results from inappropriate functioning of the autonomic nervous system. The autonomic nervous system is the part of our brain and nerves that control bodily functions over which we have no cognitive control. In order to avoid fainting when we stand, the autonomic nervous system must constrict blood vessels, increase heart rate, and increase the heart's contractility. Sometimes the autonomic nervous system malfunctions, causing inappropriate dilatation of the blood vessels and abnormal heart rates. The cause is unknown and can occur in any age, but tends to be more common in adolescents and older people. Typically, the condition occurs in healthy people without heart disease. If syncope is infrequent, no treatment may be needed. However, in some individuals syncope may be sufficiently frequent to need treatment. Lifestyle changes may be helpful. Avoid dehydration and push fluids especially when exercising on warm days. If your blood pressure runs low, extra salt may help to increase blood pressure and avoid syncope. Constantly wiggling your toes causes the leg muscles to contract and pumps blood more quickly back to your heart. Compression stockings help avoid pooling of blood in your legs. Avoid standing still for long periods of time. Most importantly, if early symptoms of lightheadedness, nausea, or unexplained sweating begin, sit down immediately to avoid passing out.

If lifestyle changes are not enough and symptoms continue, medication may be necessary. Common examples of medicines used to treat neurocardiogenic syncope include midodrine (Amatidine), mineralcorticoids (Florinef), beta-blockers, and antidepressants.

Should I take special precautions when traveling?

We want heart patients to live full and active lives. Traveling is certainly a means to do that! However, certain precautions may make your travel safer. Keep in mind the following recommendations when traveling:

- Allow extra time for travel connections when flying. Heart attacks often occur when people are stressed with time constraints.
- Watch what you eat while you travel. Salt content tends to be higher in most restaurants.
- Keep your medication with you in two separate places. If your carry-on is stolen or left behind, you will still have your pills.
- During travel, your routine will probably be interrupted. You will need to be especially careful that you take your medication on time.
- Be sure to take your diuretics, and plan extra time for their inevitable effects! The combination of no diuretics and excessive salt when you travel can precipitate heart failure quickly.

- If you have a pacemaker or defibrillator, be sure to keep your manufacturer's card with you at all times. No one can communicate with your device through a computer without knowing the specific manufacturer.
- If you fly overseas and encounter significant time change, gradually adjust the dosing intervals of your medication by two hour increments until you are back on your time schedule.
- Traveling at an altitude may require some changes in your usual activities. Symptoms of chest discomfort and shortness of breath may be more noticeable between 5000 and 7500 feet above sea level. Above 7500 feet, you should be very cautiously active, and engage in your usual walking activities slowly and gradually until you can assess the effect that altitude has on your heart.
- Consider travel insurance. Health problems occasionally arise quickly when you have heart disease, and canceling a trip will come much easier if your costs are reimbursed.

Chapter 6: Tips for Better Care

During twenty-eight years in the private practice of cardiology, I have witnessed numerous opportunities for my patients to improve their health, and avoid some of the pitfalls that may result in disastrous outcomes. Here are some tips to avoid these pitfalls:

- Try to have only one dose of any medication in your house. Having more than one dose greatly increases the likelihood for error.

- Always keep an accurate and up to date medicine list with you in your wallet or purse. Make sure that the dosage amounts and frequencies are included.

- Whenever possible, ask your physician to use electronic prescribing to your pharmacy. Legibility errors will decrease dramatically, and it's more convenient as well!

- Don't keep nitroglycerin in a tight pocket. Your body heat will markedly shorten its effectiveness.

- Always ask your doctor about possible drug interactions between your currently prescribed medication and every new medicine recommended to you.

- Don't store your medicines on the kitchen windowsill. Heat, light and air destroy many medicines.

- Always inquire about whether new symptoms you experience may be due to side effects to your medication. Examples of symptoms that are rarely considered to be side effects to drugs include cough, muscle soreness, and fainting.

- Always ask your cardiologist before stopping any medication even for brief periods. Many doctors and dentists do not understand the risks involved. This is especially true for blood thinners.

- Keep your medicines in two different locations when you travel. That way, a stolen purse will not leave you without your medication.

- Use a pill planner. This is a small box used to store all of your medication for one week at a time. A pill planner is your best protection against taking too many doses or forgetting them.

- If your medication dose is changed, re-write the directions on the pillbox. This way, the hospital staff will know the correct dose if you land in the emergency room.

- Learn to read food labels accurately and use them frequently.

- Buy and use a home blood pressure cuff on a regular basis.

- Become a compelling advocate for your own health care. Ask questions and expect answers.

Chapter 7: Facts and Fiction

"Old wives' tales" are allegedly untrue stories passed down from generation to generation, originally describing the English woman's experiences with pregnancy and child rearing. Medicine is full of such untrue perceptions, and the lives of some patients are inadvertently affected by them. Here are some of my favorites:

Fiction: Chest pain caused by heart disease is always felt in the left arm.

Fact: Chest pain caused by heart disease may be felt in the right arm, left arm, or in neither arm, and is occasionally felt in the throat and jaws.

Fiction: Chest pain is not coming from my heart if taking nitroglycerin doesn't help.

Fact: Cardiac pain is not always relieved by nitroglycerin, especially if you're having a heart attack.

Fiction: If I think I'm having a heart attack, I can get myself to the hospital safer and faster if I drive.

Fact: An electrocardiogram to diagnose your heart attack, and aspirin and nitroglycerin to treat it, are provided to you faster and safer by emergency medical services called to your home. In addition, serious and sometimes fatal cardiac rhythm disturbances can be treated en route by EMS, but can be fatal when they occur in a car.

Fiction: hypertension inevitably causes symptoms.

Fact: Hypertension usually causes symptoms only when blood pressure is very elevated and complicated by a heart attack or stroke.

Fiction: generic drugs are not good for me.

Fact: In most instances common generic drugs will save you a lot of money, and are completely equivalent to brand names. Only a few exceptions exist. For most generics, the incidence of side effects is the same as it is with brand names. Talk to your doctor about using generic drugs.

Fiction: food labels accurately describe fat and sodium content.

Fact: Although food labels are generally regarded to be accurate, watch serving sizes carefully. Stated serving sizes are typically much smaller than what most of us consume. For example, if the label quotes 100 mg of sodium in ¼ cup serving size, your sodium intake will be 400 mg if you typically consume a one cup serving.

Fiction: I can't walk very fast so exercise does me no good.

Fact: Most of the benefits from exercise come from the frequency and duration of your walking. Even a light stroll for 20 to 30 minutes repeated on most days each week will help lower your blood pressure and improve your fitness level.

Fiction: A normal electrocardiogram excludes a heart attack.

Fact: Small heart attacks and occasionally those on the bottom surface of the heart muscle may not show up on the electrocardiogram. A resting EKG is nearly worthless to exclude blockages that have not yet caused a heart attack.

Fiction: It is not necessary to share your over-the-counter medications or herbal medicines that you take each day with your doctor.

Fact: Many over the counter and herbal medicines may have an impact on your heart disease or may interact with other medicines you take. For instance, non-steroidal anti-inflammatory drugs such as ibuprofen (Advil, Motrin) may interfere with the favorable effects of aspirin, and may increase the risk of heart rupture during a heart attack.

Fiction: It is okay to stop my clopidogrel (Plavix) for a dental procedure or colonoscopy.

Fact: Stopping clopidogrel too early after placement of a stent may cause it to quickly clot closed. Never stop your Plavix without speaking first with your cardiologist.

Fiction: My high LDL cholesterol level is acceptable, because I also have a high HDL level.

Fact: A high LDL is a risk factor for having vascular disease independently of HDL. Therefore, although a high HDL is good to have, it does not negate the importance of lowering your LDL.

Fiction: Allergic reactions to medications occur shortly after they are prescribed.

Fact: You can develop an allergy to bee stings at any time in your life. Similarly, allergic reactions to medication can begin even years after you have started them.

Fiction: I should stop aspirin one to two weeks before my upcoming operation.

Fact: In most instances, aspirin does not promote enough bleeding to warrant discontinuing the drug prior to general surgery. In fact, aspirin can help reduce your chances of having a heart attack during or shortly after an operation and should usually be continued.

Fiction: Medication can usually be stopped once symptoms go away.

Fact: Very few problems with your heart can be cured by medication. In most instances, symptoms are improved and outcomes are better, but the disease will come back if medication is stopped.

Fiction: If my pills are big, I can always crush them.

Fact: Although this can be done with some medication, others such as long acting formulations can be significantly altered by crushing. Check with your pharmacist first.

Fiction: If I eat well, my cholesterol must be acceptable.

Fact: Although your cholesterol value is significantly influenced by what you eat, your genetic makeup also has a significant impact. Even people who eat exceedingly well can have dangerously high levels.

Fiction: My doctor has said nothing about my risk factors for heart disease, so they must be OK.

Fact: You are the best advocate for your own health. It is your responsibility to know your risk factors for heart disease and ask what you can do to improve them. Never assume anything if you are the victim who will pay the price.

Fiction: The nutrition label says "no cholesterol." Therefore, this food must be acceptable to eat.

Fact: Cholesterol and saturated or trans fats are different. Each of these products promotes arteriosclerosis. Therefore, you must avoid all three to lower your risk.

Chapter 8: Glossary

Ablation: A procedure using a hot tipped catheter to destroy unwanted electrical tissue in the heart.

Angioplasty: A procedure to open up a blocked blood vessel with a balloon-tipped catheter.

Aortic insufficiency: A leaky aortic valve that allows blood pumped into the aorta to wash back into the left ventricle.

Anticoagulant: Blood thinners.

Aortic stenosis: A stiff aortic valve that cannot open to allow the exit of blood from the left ventricle to the body.

Aortic valve: The valve located between the left ventricle and aorta that must open to allow blood to be pumped to the body.

Arteriolosclerosis: Hardening of the arteries.

Atrioventricular node (AV node): a small electrical structure midway down the heart that collects electrical impulses from the upper chambers and distributes them to the lower chambers.

Atrium (pleural: atria): the upper chambers of the heart that receive incoming blood.

Coronary arteries: The three blood vessels that supply the heart muscle with blood.

CT angiogram: An x-ray picture of the heart and its blood vessels.

Diuretics: water pills.

Edema: swelling due to fluid retention.

Embolism: A blood clot that forms in one location and travels to another location in the body.

Ejection fraction: The percentage of blood that is ejected from the heart with every heartbeat. The normal value is 55 – 65%.

Enzymes: Chemicals contained within the heart cells that spill into the blood stream if heart muscle damage has occurred.

HDL cholesterol: The "good" cholesterol.

Hemoglobin A1c: A blood test that measures how well diabetes is controlled.

Hypertension: High blood pressure.

Inferior vena cava: The large blood vessel that collects blood from the lower half of the body and returns it to the right atrium.

LDL cholesterol: The "bad" cholesterol.

Leads: The wires that connect a pacemaker or defibrillator with the heart.

Left anterior descending coronary artery: The main blood vessel that supplies the front surface of the heart and septum with blood.

Left circumflex coronary artery: The main blood vessel that supplies the back surface of the heart muscle with blood.

Left main coronary artery: a short blood vessel to the heart that gives rise to the left anterior descending and left circumflex coronary arteries.

Mitral insufficiency: a leaky mitral valve that allows blood entering into the left ventricle to wash back into the left atrium.

Mitral stenosis: A stiff mitral valve that cannot open to allow blood to enter from the left atrium the left ventricle.

Mitral valve: The valve lying between the left atrium and left ventricle.

Myocardial infarction: A heart attack.

Nitroglycerin: A medication taken under the tongue to relieve chest pain.

Plaque: A build up of cholesterol, calcium, and scar tissue that blocks a blood vessel.

Prognosis: The outcome of a disease over time.

Pulmonary valve: The valve located between the right ventricle and pulmonary arteries that opens to allow blood to get to the lungs.

Right coronary artery: The blood vessel that supplies blood to the right and bottom surface of the heart.

Septum: The wall that divides the lower two chambers of the heart, the right and left ventricles.

Sinus node: The spark plug in the upper right atrium that provides the electrical stimuli to the heart.

Sleep apnea: A condition during sleep when breathing stops due to obstruction in the airway.

Sodium: Salt.

Sphygmomanometer: A cuff to measure blood pressure.

Stent: A metal mesh device placed in a blood vessel after an angioplasty to keep the vessel open.

Superior vena cava: The large vein that collects blood from the upper half of the body and delivers it to the right atrium.

Syncope: A brief, temporary loss of consciousness.

Thrombolytic drugs: Clot-busting drugs to open up a blood vessel obstructed by clot.

Thrombosis: A blood clot.

Tricuspid valve: The valve located between the right atrium and right ventricle.

Triglycerides: fatty substances in the blood that increase the risk of heart attack and stroke.

Ventricle: The lower chambers of the heart that pump blood out of the body.

Chapter 9: Guide to abbreviations

ACE	angiotensin-converting enzyme
ACEI	angiotensin-converting enzyme inhibitor
b.i.d.	twice daily
ECG	electrocardiogram
EF	the ejection fraction
EKG	electrocardiogram
F.D.A.	the Federal Food and Drug Administration
INR	international normalized ratio
IV	intravenous
KG	kilogram
LDL	low density lipoprotein
MG	milligram
M. I.	Myocardial infarction (heart attack)
ml	milliliter
OTC	over-the-counter
qd	once daily
PCI	percutaneous coronary intervention (angioplasty)
PTCA	angioplasty
q.i.d.	4 times daily
t.i.d.	3 times daily

About the Authors

Twenty eight years ago, Dr. Westveer co-founded the Northpointe Heart Center in southeast Michigan, a busy specialty clinic that has now grown to thirteen cardiologists engaged in the evaluation and treatment of heart disease. In addition, he has helped shape the Departments of Cardiology at William Beaumont Hospital in Royal Oak and Troy, Michigan for nearly two decades. The Beaumont Hospitals system is currently amongst the largest cardiology providers in the country and have been named regularly in the U.S. News and World Report's top fifteen hospitals in cardiac care. Dr. Westveer served as vice-chief of cardiology at William Beaumont in Royal Oak, Michigan for ten years before transferring to the Troy-based hospital, where he is currently department chairman. At Troy, he led the development of a full service cardiology division engaged in cardiac intervention, electrophysiology and cardiac surgery. He has been a driving force on hospital administrative committees, regional health care advisory committees, and was an active member of the Beaumont Board of Directors for over five years. He is the author of over 50 publications relating to heart disease and has published eight books and book chapters describing the evaluation and management of heart disease for physicians.

Sandra Jordan is an educator engaged in the creation and management of Montessori schools for children. In her role, she has emphasized and perfected her need to communicate accurately and passionately to parents yet maintain the simplicity needed to talk directly and effectively with children. In the medical field, the enemy of sharing information with patients lies in the complexity and volume of medical information available from ever-growing sources. Every page of information shared in this book was first shared with Ms. Jordan. Her insight, common sense, and desire for simplicity in the explanations and vocabulary we selected played a vital role. Ms. Jordan's goal is to convey information that is appropriate, understandable, and meaningful.

BUY A SHARE OF THE FUTURE IN YOUR COMMUNITY

These certificates make great holiday, graduation and birthday gifts that can be personalized with the recipient's name. The cost of one S.H.A.R.E. or one square foot is $54.17. The personalized certificate is suitable for framing and will state the number of shares purchased and the amount of each share, as well as the recipient's name. The home that you participate in "building" will last for many years and will continue to grow in value.

Here is a sample SHARE certificate:

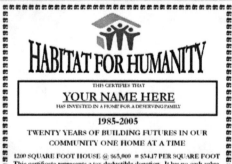

HABITAT FOR HUMANITY

THIS CERTIFIES THAT

YOUR NAME HERE

HAS INVESTED IN A HOME FOR A DESERVING FAMILY

1985-2005

TWENTY YEARS OF BUILDING FUTURES IN OUR COMMUNITY ONE HOME AT A TIME

1200 SQUARE FOOT HOUSE @ $65,000 = $54.17 PER SQUARE FOOT
This certificate represents a tax deductible donation. It has no cash value.

YES, I WOULD LIKE TO HELP!

I support the work that Habitat for Humanity does and I want to be part of the excitement! As a donor, I will receive periodic updates on your construction activities but, more importantly, I know my gift will help a family in our community realize the dream of homeownership. **I would like to SHARE in your efforts against substandard housing in my community!** *(Please print below)*

PLEASE SEND ME _____ SHARES at $54.17 EACH = $ $_____

In Honor Of: _____

Occasion: (Circle One)   *HOLIDAY   BIRTHDAY   ANNIVERSARY*

 OTHER: _____

Address of Recipient: _____

Gift From: _____ *Donor Address:* _____

Donor Email: _____

I AM ENCLOSING A CHECK FOR $ $_____ PAYABLE TO HABITAT FOR HUMANITY OR PLEASE CHARGE MY VISA OR MASTERCARD *(CIRCLE ONE)*

Card Number _____ Expiration Date: _____

Name as it appears on Credit Card _____ Charge Amount $ _____

Signature _____

Billing Address _____

Telephone # Day _____ Eve _____

PLEASE NOTE: Your contribution is tax-deductible to the fullest extent allowed by law.
Habitat for Humanity • P.O. Box 1443 • Newport News, VA 23601 • 757-596-5553
www.HelpHabitatforHumanity.org

LaVergne, TN USA
02 November 2009
162816LV00010B/1/P